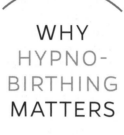

WHY
HYPNO-
BIRTHING
MATTERS

Pinter & Martin Why it Matters

There is more information available on giving birth and raising children than ever before. With each new scientific advance or fad, more questions arise. The Why It Matters series seeks to steer a course through this sea of information, and offer succinct, balanced and evidence-based introductions to a wide range of subjects, giving readers a firm framework from which to make confident, informed decisions of their own.

Spring 2015

1   Why the Politics of Breastfeeding Matter
2   Why Hypnobirthing Matters
3   Why Doulas Matter

Autumn 2015

4   Why Pre-Conception and Pregnancy Nutrition Matters
5   Why Breastfeeding Matters
6   Why Baby-Led Weaning Matters

2016 and beyond

Why Your Baby's Sleep Matters | Why Perinatal Depression Matters | Why Babywearing Matters | Why Your Birth Experience Matters | Why VBAC Matters | Why Attachment Parenting Matters | Why Home Birth Matters | Why Midwives Matter | Why Fathers Matter | Why Tests in Pregnancy Matter *and many more*

for the latest titles, please visit
pinterandmartin.com/why-it-matters

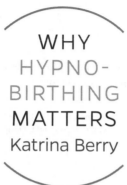

WHY
HYPNO-
BIRTHING
MATTERS
Katrina Berry

pinter
&
martin

Why Hypnobirthing Matters (Pinter & Martin Why It Matters: 2)

First published by Pinter & Martin Ltd 2015

© 2015 Katrina Berry

ISBN 978-1-78066-505-4
Also available as ebook

Pinter & Martin Why It Matters ISSN 2056-8657

Series editor: Susan Last
Index: Helen Bilton
Proofreader: Debbie Kennett

British Library Cataloguing-in-Publication Data
A catalogue record for this book is available from the British Library.

Set in Minion

Printed and bound in the UK by Ashford Colour Press Ltd, Gosport, Hampshire

This book has been printed on paper that is sourced and harvested from sustainable forests and is FSC accredited.

Pinter & Martin Ltd
6 Effra Parade
London SW2 1PS

pinterandmartin.com

Contents

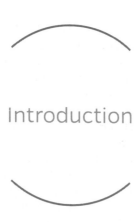

Introduction

This book is for you if you're pregnant, hoping to be pregnant, know someone who's pregnant or work within the area of pregnancy and birth. It's for those who are interested in how our minds work, the power of the mind over the body and how we can train it to work for us. My aim is to show how and why hypnosis for birth has become so popular and why it matters: for mothers, fathers, babies and those who support them through pregnancy and birth.

Hypnobirthing is a process, not a method. 'Hypnobirthing' has simply become the most recognisable term for the use of hypnosis and hypnotherapy to help to improve the experience of childbirth. You'll notice that I use hypnobirthing and HypnoBirthing interchangeably within the book. I'm not trying to confuse you, I just want to highlight that they are the same thing. This book is not about a particular 'method' of hypnosis for birth; the philosophy and principles of all hypnosis for birth courses are the same and they all have the same goal. At the end of the book we'll take a look at the main hypnobirthing courses and books currently available in the UK, with contributions from the founders of each programme.

Let's get one thing straight right away. There is no one right way to give birth; every baby's birth is unique. Hypnobirthing is not just for those planning a natural birth. A 'hypno birth' is not necessarily at home, in water, in the dark, surrounded by whale music. Of course there are many women who choose that for themselves, but there are also those who give birth in birthing centres and labour wards, and those whose babies come unexpectedly in the strangest of places. Some babies and mothers need help and, thankfully, in the UK we have a wonderful maternity system that offers medical assistance. Hypnobirthing helps in all these scenarios.

We'll split the word HypnoBirthing up and look at the 'hypno' part – the history of using hypnosis for birth and how it has developed, taking a look at the rationale for its use and how it works. We'll explore 'birthing' and you'll gain an understanding of how the female body is designed to give birth when uninterrupted, and learn how you can create conditions conducive to calm, comfortable childbirth.

Sadly fear, anxiety and ignorance about natural childbirth are prevalent in our society and one of the best ways I know to counteract the horror stories so often told of childbirth is to share empowering and uplifting stories. I'm honoured to share with you stories from many people who've used hypnobirthing in a wide range of circumstances. You'll hear, in their own words, how this approach helped them through pregnancy, birth and beyond.

Hypnobirthing does not guarantee an easy or pain-free birth – nothing can guarantee that. There are many things, externally and internally, individually and culturally, that can impede us. However, with preparation and information we can optimise the functioning of our bodies and minds so that the welcoming of your baby is a calm, joyous occasion. This is what HypnoBirthing offers to everyone that does it.

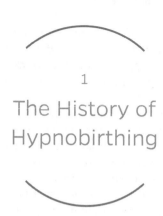

1
The History of Hypnobirthing

The term hypnobirthing is used to describe the use of hypnosis and hypnotherapy to help improve the experience of childbirth. The origins of most current hypnobirthing programmes can be traced back to the pioneering work of British obstetrician Dr Grantly Dick-Read, who attended a birth in 1912 that would change his life:

I had ploughed through mud and rain on my bicycle between two and three in the morning down Whitechapel Road.... Having groped and stumbled my way up a dark staircase, I opened the door of a room about ten feet square. There was a pool of water lying on the floor, the window was broken, rain was pouring in, the bed had no proper covering and was kept up at one end by a sugar box. My patient lay covered only with sacks and an old black skirt. The room was lit by one candle stuck in the top of a beer bottle on the mantleshelf. A neighbour had brought in a jug of water and a basin; I had to provide my own soap and towel. In spite of this setting – which even thirty years ago was a disgrace to any civilised country – I soon became conscious of a quiet kindliness in the atmosphere.

In due course, the baby was born. There was no fuss or noise. Everything seemed to have been carried out according to an ordered plan. There was only one slight dissension: I tried to persuade my patient to let me put the mask over her face and give her some chloroform when the head appeared and the dilation of the passages was obvious. She, however, resented the suggestion and firmly but kindly refused to take this help. It was the first time in my short experience that I had ever been refused when offering chloroform. As I was about to leave some time later I asked her why it was that she would not use the mask. She did not answer at once, but looked from the old woman who had been assisting to the window through which was bursting the first light of dawn; and then shyly she turned to me and said: 'It didn't hurt. It wasn't meant to, was it, doctor?'

For weeks and months afterwards, as I sat with women in labour, women who appeared to be in the terror and agony of childbirth, that sentence came drumming back into my ears… finally, even through my orthodox and conservative mind, I began to see the light. I began to realise that there was no law in nature and no design that could justify the pain of childbirth. Not many years afterwards the war took me to foreign lands. There I witnessed women having their babies in the most natural and apparently painless manner, but I also saw those who suffered pain and to whom the birth of their child was an experience horrible to remember…

It was very difficult to explain why one should suffer and another be apparently free from pain... It slowly dawned on me, however, that it was the peacefulness of a relatively painless labour that distinguished it most clearly from the others. There was calm, it seemed almost faith, in the normal and natural outcome of childbirth.

Childbirth Without Fear, Pinter & Martin, 2013

Based on what he was observing, Dick-Read postulated that the fear experienced by a woman in childbirth caused blood to be diverted away from her uterus in order to be used by other muscles to enable her to escape from danger. The result of this was to deprive the uterus of oxygen, preventing it from carrying out its intended function without pain. This phenomenon he called 'the fear-tension-pain syndrome of childbirth'.

Dr Dick-Read believed that if a woman were able to eliminate fear, her uterus would return to its normal function, thus eliminating the pain. Concluding that fear and tension were responsible for 95 per cent of labour pain, he suggested this could be eliminated through relaxation techniques. While he staunchly refused the suggestion that he was using hypnosis, this was at a time when hypnosis was largely misunderstood. We now have a clearer understanding of the science of our mind and the benefits of hypnosis – we know that not only is hypnosis a wonderful tool for relaxation, but it is also effective in changing a person's thought patterns and therefore helps eliminate fear and anxiety going into labour.

Building a woman's confidence and trust in her body's ability to birth allows her to be able to step gracefully out of the way and allow her body and baby to do what they know how to do.

The development of hypnobirthing

Throughout its history, hypnotherapy has been used in relation to childbirth. James Braid, commonly regarded as the founder of hypnotherapy, reports a case in which hypnotic suggestion was used to induce labour for medical reasons in 1858. However, the largest and most systematic use of hypnosis for childbirth took place in the Soviet Union at the start of the 20th century. Tens of thousands of women received hypnosis and a surprising amount of data was collected on its use. In order to make it accessible to a wider audience (again the term hypnosis was misunderstood and mistrusted) the term 'psychoprophylaxis' was used (meaning the psychological prevention of pain and anxiety during childbirth). Psychoprophylaxis strove to eliminate the pain of childbirth through education about the physiological process of birth, through the trained relaxation response to uterine contractions, and through patterned breathing intended to both increase oxygenation and interfere with the transmission of pain signals from the uterus to the cerebral cortex.

It was this that the French obstetrician Dr Fernand Lamaze witnessed when he visited Moscow in the 1940s; he was so impressed that, after he returned to France, he devoted the rest of his life to promoting the 'Lamaze method', which he based on what he'd seen in Russia. In the early years, Lamaze was unabashedly about self-hypnosis, but he too dropped the term after meeting resistance and misunderstanding. The Lamaze method gained popularity in the United States after Marjorie Karmel wrote about her experiences in her 1959 book, *Thank You, Dr. Lamaze*.

Also in the US, in the 1940s, Dr Robert Bradley became a natural childbirth proponent, coming to many of the same conclusions that Dr Grantly Dick-Read had before him. From Dr Bradley's work came his book *Husband-Coached Childbirth* and Bradley childbirth classes. Dr Bradley was very interested in hypnosis and originally promoted his 'method' as using hypnosis. Eventually, however, the emphasis on hypnosis was dropped and the focus became 'deep relaxation' instead.

Dr Philip Magonet, president and founder of the Medical Hypnosis Association in the 1950s, believed that 'the time will come when hypnotherapy in antenatal clinics will be regarded as just as important as carrying out pelvic measurements, blood pressure reading and urine examination'. Indeed, during the 1960s there was a good deal of interest in self-hypnosis for birth and a number of studies were published supporting the effectiveness of hypnosis in obstetrics, reporting high rates (58–93 per cent) of women giving birth with hypnosis as their sole form of pain relief.

The origin of the term 'hypnobirthing' in around 1987 is accredited to Michelle Leclaire O'Neill in the USA, who has written several books on the subject of childbirth including *Hypnobirthing: the Original Method*. Also in the USA, Marie Mongan wrote *Hypnobirthing – A Celebration of Life* in 1989 and created 'The Mongan Method', which gained recognition further afield as word-of-mouth recommendations increased and it began to be taught in the UK.

Natal Hypnotherapy was the first hypnosis for birth programme developed solely in the UK to work alongside the NHS guidelines for birth. Maggie Howell developed the programme as a result of using basic self-hypnosis, Neuro-Linguistic Programming (NLP) and instinctive birthing for the birth of her first child. To understand more about what she had actually done, and how the hypnosis had worked, she trained to become a clinical hypnotherapist and in 2000 created the first Natal Hypnotherapy CD.

The last 15 years have seen great advances in the field of hypnosis for birth, with many studies into its effectiveness and more programmes evolving from the original teaching. Most people, however, still find out about hypnobirthing through word of mouth – they then look into it and find that there is a wide choice of courses, books and CDs. It can be confusing for a newly expectant couple or those working in birth. There are currently five main methods of hypnosis for birth available in the UK: KG Hypnobirthing, Mindful Mamma, The Mongan Method, Natal Hypnotherapy and the Wise Hippo birthing programme. Ultimately there's very little difference between them; they vary slightly in content, length and delivery, but they all have the same goals and philosophy and use the work of Dr Grantly Dick-Read as their foundation.

While early approaches to the use of hypnosis for birth emphasised using hypnotic techniques as a pain management tool, hypnobirthing programmes are now much more comprehensive. Often a complete antenatal course, all of the hypnosis for birth courses and books educate women and their partners about nature's design of the birthing body and how best to create conditions conducive to natural birthing. Couples are taught how beliefs and thoughts affect our nervous system and how they can help or hinder the birth process. Facing fears and releasing concerns, through hypnosis, allows a couple to approach their birth with calm confidence. Far from being 'hippy trippy', hypnobirthing programmes are rooted in science and all methods pride themselves on encouraging evidence-based birth practice. They will often teach parents-to-be about the NHS health system, the roles of midwives, obstetricians and doctors, and give them the confidence to navigate hospital policies and guidelines to make informed decisions. Most courses will also look at physical as well as emotional and psychological preparation for birth.

To help you get a sense of any similarities and differences

between the methods available I put some 'frequently asked questions' to the founders of each so, for the first time you can hear from them all together in their own words (see page 135).

Hypnobirthing courses are predominantly still taught by private practitioners who have been trained in a specific approach and bring their own experience and skills to their teaching. The growth in popularity of hypnobirthing, and the increased awareness of its effectiveness, means you'll now find an increasing number of NHS health trusts throughout the UK offering hypnobirthing. Sadly lack of funding means the cost of the courses can vary, as can the length and content of the course. Typically a full hypnobirthing course will be 12 hours to cover all areas of antenatal preparation; chapter 5 will look at what you can expect from hypnobirthing.

Since the 1960s there has been a huge rise in the availability of pharmacological pain relief, particularly epidurals, along with an increase in surgical intervention. There is now, however, a growing recognition that effective relief of pain does not necessarily equate with women feeling satisfied with their birth experience. One of the most comprehensive studies on hypnosis for pain relief in childbirth was conducted in 2007 by Brown and Hammond and found that the hypnotised group of women were about half as likely to require pharmaceutical pain relief during childbirth as those women giving birth without hypnosis. More specifically 62 per cent of hypnotised women did not require analgesia, compared to only 26 per cent of non-hypnotised women.

At the time of writing, we are awaiting the results of the SHIP study (Self-Hypnosis for Intrapartum Pain management), the most recent, and largest, randomised controlled trial of first-time mothers in the UK, carried out by Professor Soo Downe to add to the evidence base on the effectiveness of hypnosis as a pain and stress reliever for birth. In the interim Professor Downe has said, 'Along with other techniques that women use to help them to work with the processes of pregnancy, labour and birth, the reports from practice indicate that many of those who use hypnosis find that it supports them in achieving their aims, even when things don't always go according to plan. It is therefore important that pregnant women can have access to learning about how to achieve an hypnotic state.'

Whatever the SHIP study concludes, it's worth remembering how hard it is to prove the effectiveness of something that has so many variables. Reviews of research studies show just how complex it is to study hypnosis and self-hypnosis. Some studies are unclear about whether women offered hypnosis were also shown how to use self-hypnosis during labour, and the amount and timing of preparation is often varied, so it's hard to get qualitative statistics. Cochrane reviews are systematic reviews of primary research in human health care and health policy, and are internationally recognised as the highest standard in evidence-based health care. The Cochrane review into complementary and alternative therapies for pain management in labour, published in 2006, found evidence to suggest that hypnosis:

- decreases the need for pharmacological pain relief
- reduces induction and augmentation of labour
- shortens the length of labour
- increases the incidence of spontaneous vaginal birth
- is associated with improved maternal well-being and satisfaction and
- is beneficial to neonatal outcomes

We're reaching a tipping point in the world of birth; there's growing dissatisfaction in the medicalisation of childbirth and the possible consequences. There is a resurgence of interest in a non-invasive, non-medicated approach to birth. There's a groundswell of social media groups, grassroots movements and formal organisations vociferously supporting a woman's choice. There are celebrities and well-known women talking in the media about birthing their babies calmly and confidently using hypnobirthing. The studies and research are backing up what we've known for decades and, although it's slow, there is a growing recognition of the benefits of using hypnosis for antenatal preparation and birth.

Perhaps, finally, we're not too far away from Magonet's vision of sixty years ago.

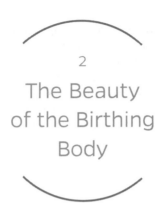

2

The Beauty
of the Birthing
Body

*When birth is undisturbed, our birthing hormones can
take us into ecstasy – outside (ec) our usual state (stasis) –
so that we enter motherhood awakened and transformed.*

Dr Sarah Buckley, *Gentle Birth, Gentle Mothering*

Since Dr Grantly Dick-Read wrote about his observations in
birthing women and postulated about the fear-tension-pain
cycle, we have, over the last fifty years, done a great deal of
research into what happens to a woman's body during pregnancy
and birth. We now know that his theory was absolutely right,
and, as we are such rational creatures, having a scientific
understanding of how a woman's body is designed to give birth
is the best place to start. It astonishes me that we are not taught
more of this in school, or even in other antenatal courses. To
understand your body is to appreciate it, and to appreciate it is
to start to rebuild trust and confidence in your body's ability to
birth. What I am about to describe is an undisturbed birth, by
which I mean birth as it plays out when it starts naturally and

unfolds without intervention, just as nature intends.

Birth is all about hormones and muscles, and when you understand the exquisite cocktail of hormones that fuels birth you're better able to create the optimal conditions to bring them about. A hormone is a chemical released into the bloodstream to send a message to another part of the body. It is often referred to as a 'chemical messenger'. As a woman I've been well aware of their power since puberty. I consider myself a rational and pragmatic person, and yet once a month I can turn into a mushy-brained, emotionally-charged demon who will just as likely jump down your throat as go hide under a duvet. If you're a woman reading this, you may be all too familiar with the power hormones have over our bodies and minds; as a man reading this, if you've lived with a woman you'll probably be aware too – if not a little bewildered and in awe!

From the second of conception, our female body knows how to handle this miracle of life. The right hormones are secreted at the right time, the nourishment and support of the baby during pregnancy is ensured, the cartilage of the cervix softens, the ligaments become more flexible. Long before labour oestrogen and progesterone start to set the scene for birth, beginning to prepare and reorganise other hormone systems. Levels increase dramatically during pregnancy: the dominant type of pregnancy oestrogen, estriol, rises by more than one thousand times with a surge before the onset of labour.

Despite all the research there are still some fundamental processes of childbirth that are not fully understood. For instance, we're not 100 per cent certain what causes the onset of birth. Current thinking suggests that many factors are likely to be involved, with communication between mother and baby to ensure both are ready for the journey. This is a partnership after all, and mother and baby make the journey together. Your baby is very involved in their own birth.

We do know that the length of gestation varies for every woman and baby and generally falls somewhere between 37 and 42 weeks, although I've known a fair number of 43 and 44-week babies. When hoping for a natural birth the most important step is to allow the process to start naturally. This way you know both your baby and your body are ready. One of the main understandings we currently have is that when babies are ready for life in the outside world they produce a protein that enters the amniotic fluid. This protein acts as the green light, a 'good to go' sign that your brain recognises and so starts the birth process, with the main hormonal player in childbirth, oxytocin.

Forget diamonds, oxytocin is a girl's best friend...

In 1906 the English researcher Sir Henry Dale discovered a substance in the pituitary gland that could speed up the birthing process. He named it oxytocin, from the Greek words for 'swift' and 'childbirth labour'. We now have a greater understanding of the wide range of roles oxytocin plays and there are many books solely dedicated to this hormone, which gives you an indication of how powerful and important it is to us as a species. It has been called the hormone of love, the shy hormone, the cuddle hormone, the moral molecule, the hormone of altruism, the hormone of empathy, the hormone of forgetting oneself, the 'trust me' drug – you get the gist.

Oxytocin is the hormone you produce when you fall in love, when you have an orgasm, when you meet your baby, when you breastfeed, when you're with close friends and family, when you feel closely connected to someone. It is also the most powerful uterotonic hormone and its release is associated with the surges of birth in all mammalian species.

That rise in oestrogen before birth increases the number of uterine oxytocin receptors within the uterus in late pregnancy, effectively wiring up the uterus for coordinated muscle activity (surges or contractions) during birth. Oxytocin is thought to be the prime initiator of these rhythmic surges in the uterine muscles once your baby is ready. Often a woman's body will warm up for days or even weeks before birth, with these muscles practising working together so that when the baby is ready they can slowly get into their rhythm as your body finds its own momentum. This is where the muscles come into their own.

Some interesting facts about oxytocin

- Oxytocin release can be hindered by a stressful environment, as fight-or-flight hormones inhibit oxytocin.
- Oxytocin is released in pulses of about 90 seconds, and lasts in the body for about three minutes. Its effects can last up to three hours.
- Oxytocin contributes to the healing of tissues.
- Rhythmical stroking of the skin (at about 40 beats per minute) releases oxytocin – five minutes of stroking leads to a reduction in blood pressure for up to three hours
- Eating good food produces oxytocin.
- Oxytocin has direct effects on brain growth, especially the neo-cortex of the newborn.
- Oxytocin is released during orgasm for both men and women. Orgasm has a host of physical and emotional health benefits, so don't forget to give your partner the nudge now and again!
- An epidural impacts the effects of oxytocin by blocking the transmission up the spinal cord. However, since oxytocin also increases your pain threshold, an epidural may not be needed. The highest peak of oxytocin in a

---

woman's lifetime is right after her baby is born, but before the placenta is delivered – we can maximise the hormone's potential by placing baby skin-to-skin with mum and leaving the two undisturbed during this time.

- Skin-to-skin contact increases oxytocin release.
  – whether it's mother and baby right after birth, dad massaging his infant, or mum and dad holding hands.
- Oxytocin helps your body use nutrients through digestion, and aids in transferring those to the baby during pregnancy and as nutrients into breastmilk.
- Oxytocin is also released during breastfeeding, which increases the activity in the gastrointestinal tract so the mother uses calories more efficiently.
- Aside from its reproductive roles, oxytocin is released when sharing a meal with a friend, hugging someone you care about, and even when petting your dog. So if you're feeling down, spend some quality time with a good friend and hug those you care about and love.

There is no other organ quite like the uterus. If men had such an organ, they would brag about it. So should we.

Ina May Gaskin

The muscles of the uterus are extremely powerful and made up of three layers. The outer longitudinal muscles go up around the top of the baby, the middle layer is interspersed with blood vessels, keeping the uterus replenished with fresh oxygenated blood, and the innermost layer of horizontal bands of muscles encircle your baby and come down to form what looks a little like a bottleneck. That bottleneck is your cervix, a powerful band of muscles that holds the uterus tightly closed until birth begins.

Before pregnancy, the uterus is a hollow muscular organ

the shape and size of an inverted pear. The layers of muscle fibres are powerful yet flexible, allowing the uterus to expand during pregnancy to roughly the size of a watermelon (if there is just the one baby inside!) – most of the time without you even being aware of it. The uterus also functions painlessly in its normal functioning at times other than during pregnancy and birth. During menstruation, the uterus contracts, and the cervix opens to allow the lining to pass. Most women will not experience pain during this process. (Don't worry if you do, we'll come back to this). Although the uterus is not directly involved in sexual activity, it does undergo changes during sexual excitement. When a woman is sexually aroused, the uterus lifts upward, increases in size and remains enlarged until orgasm or until stimulation stops. The uterus contracts painlessly during orgasm.

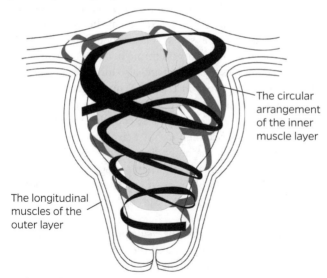

The circular arrangement of the inner muscle layer

The longitudinal muscles of the outer layer

The circular, longitudinal and spiralling muscle fibres of the uterus.

Every muscle in the body functions by contraction and release. No healthy muscle, going about its normal function, hurts. Normal functions such as walking, flexing a bicep or the beating of a healthy heart do not hurt. The muscles of the uterus are normal too.

When the uterus is in surge the outer and innermost layers of muscle are working together as a pair. As the outer muscles tighten, the inner muscles release. It's this release that allows the cervix, that bottleneck, to thin and open – what the clinical world call 'stage one' of labour. This process of the cervix thinning and opening can take time, particularly the first time a woman gives birth, as your body finds its momentum and the baby moves into a good position (if it hasn't already).

The cervix is ordinarily rather cartilagenous, quite firm, rather like your nose. The combination of relaxin (a hormone that 'does exactly what it says on the tin', it relaxes tissues) and prostaglandins allow it to soften so that by the time your baby is ready, your cervix is as soft as your earlobe and better able to thin and open for baby to pass through. Oxytocin stimulates the uterine muscles to contract and also increases production of prostaglandins, which increase the contractions further.

Increased levels of stretch receptors in the uterus trigger oxytocin that is released in pulses, coordinating beautifully with the release of beta-endorphin. Scientists working on the effects of opiates on the body discovered endorphins (that's how they got their name, it's short for endogenous morphine). They found that endorphins are up to 200 times more potent than morphine and that they are produced naturally from the pituitary gland in the brain.

Endorphins suppress the synaptic activity that is responsible for sensing pain and they also create a tranquil, amnesiac state. Some researchers believe that endorphins are the reward we get for performing reproductive functions such as mating and birthing; that is, the endorphin fix keeps us having sex and having babies. Beta-endorphin and oxytocin work synergistically in pacing the birth process: very high levels of beta-endorphin cause the oxytocin level to reduce and contractions will slow down slightly. Overall this positive feedback loop allows the surges to slowly build in frequency, length and intensity, with the cervix softening, thinning and opening and endorphin levels steadily increasing.

Back to uterine activity during menstruation and the good news if you've suffered with painful periods in the past. While the uterine muscles are essentially doing the same work, the hormonal cocktail is much stronger during childbirth thanks to those increased levels of stretch receptors and increased levels of oxytocin and endorphins. This is, I believe, why we naturally seek out endorphins during menstruation (when we don't have the benefit of those extra oxytocin receptors) – exercise, warm baths, chocolate, wine, orgasm – these are all great producers of endorphins. They can all be helpful during labour too, but the design of the birthing body has already taken care of this need for extra endorphins and will keep topping up levels as baby comes closer.

The build-up of surges means they take up more of your attention, and the increased oxytocin and endorphins naturally encourage a woman to want to withdraw from everyday life and go somewhere safe (without this instinct women would be giving birth all over the place!) and focus on their coming baby.

There is so much focus on the contractions (surges, or rushes), that the rests in between can be forgotten and they are well worth remembering. I've been in awe, sitting with a woman in labour, watching the intensity and power of a surge, aware of how all-encompassing it can be as she breathes with and through it, it comes to a peak and starts to roll away as her body softens and lets go… and then the body rests and it's as if it were never there. There is complete focus and power, and then complete rest; the body's innate way of conserving energy.

To push or not to push…

Once the cervix is fully open a combination of the uterine surges and some pressure from the abdominal muscles, along with the baby moving herself and the rhythmic, wave-like motions of the birth path itself (a bit like peristalsis in digestion), pushes the baby out of the body. The clinical world call this 'stage two' of birth and it's where the question of whether to push, or not to push, arises.

One of the most vivid examples that shows that birth is not a conscious effort – by which I mean you cannot will it to happen – is that there are documented cases of women in comas giving birth naturally, vaginally. Take a moment to think about that…

There is no need to forcibly push a baby out of your body; your body and baby will take care of this all by themselves. This is in direct opposition to what you will have seen on TV and in the movies, where a red-faced, sweating woman will grasp onto something, anything, put her chin to her chest (she's probably lying on a bed!), take a deep breath, hold it and *puuuuush!* This is called the Valsalva manoeuvre and thankfully studies now show what we've known all along – it's counter-productive. It can reduce oxygen levels, increase carbon dioxide levels, cause every muscle in your body to tighten and it's exhausting.

When, however, every cell of your being is telling you to push, you want to work with your body and baby effectively. This 'urge to push' is common: renowned French obstetrician Michel Odent calls it 'the naturally expulsive reflex' and it is your body pushing anyway. Tuning into your body and instinct means you can work with it in a much gentler and yet more effective way. Hypnobirthing teaches a woman to breathe her baby out. This is not some namby-pamby limp breathing, but really using the power of your breath and intention to work with your baby and your body and all be moving in the same direction, at the same time. I should also say that there are some women who don't experience that urge to push and have been completely taken aback to reach down and feel their baby emerging. This again illustrates the fact that you don't *have* to do anything.

As the baby moves down through the pelvis (the joints and ligaments of which have been loosened through the production of relaxin through pregnancy), the birth path itself helps manoeuvre the baby down and they can get in on the act too. Don't be fooled; these babies are robust beings, fully involved in their own births. Some babies have been seen to push off the top of the uterus with their feet to help propel themselves down and out!

Non-forceful pushing means working with the surges and resting in between – this process of baby moving down and back slightly helps prepare both baby and mother for baby's eventual emergence into the world. The surges help a baby mould to her mother (you'll probably already be aware that a baby's skull isn't fully fused at birth; the plates of the skull, called fontanels, overlap and align themselves to shape the head for easy birth) and enable the tissues of the perineum to stretch. Gloria Lemay, a private birth attendant and doula trainer in Canada, has likened a birthing mother to a sculptress. We'd expect Michelangelo to take time when crafting a work of art, and allowing a baby to come in her own time has much to recommend it.

As a baby emerges oxytocin levels rise higher than ever before. This is Mother Nature's way of ensuring that a mother falls in love with her child; it's the height of bonding and attachment, so that in a couple of weeks' time when baby needs feeding in the middle of the night mum will do so rather than ignoring her. The oxytocin rush helps to bring milk to the breast – the baby arrives ready to breastfeed and will often latch on almost immediately after birth. This in turn brings about more oxytocin, more feelings of love and attachment and, importantly, keeps the surges productive for the placenta to be expelled and for everything to close up and retract – what is known as the 'third stage' of birth.

And so it comes full circle: oxytocin starts birth, establishes and maintains the momentum of surges in both muscles and hormones to bring baby forth, and then closes the circle and physical process.

What an intricate and intelligent design; but then with something as important as the continuation of the human species, wouldn't we expect it to be? It may be that you've never heard birth talked about in such a way. In fact our society seems to view birth as fundamentally flawed and a process that needs medical help to get started and keep going, saving women from their dysfunctional bodies.

Why is this? Let's take a look now at what could prevent birth playing out in the way in which it is designed.

winners, and as human beings we're naturally inclined to be more interested in a dramatic story – that's why soap operas are so popular. So we get super-speedy births (sitcoms and soap operas are 22 minutes long, so it needs to happen quickly): a woman suddenly clutches her belly as she feels an overwhelming sensation out of nowhere and then starts panicking. We get the all-too-familiar portrayal of a woman lying on her back, legs often propped up in stirrups, pushing until her face is purple and screaming in pain. We are taught to believe that birth is an inevitably painful and unpleasant experience; that it is a medical event that must be endured.

As if those dramatised versions of childbirth aren't bad enough, we then have to face the negative birth stories we hear from our own mothers, relatives and friends: even perfect strangers feel they need to warn you how awful it can be. Right from childhood we are bombarded with images that teach us that childbirth is agony. Women who have had children often do nothing to help expectant mothers. It is a very strange thing that a high percentage of women delight in recalling their own 'dreadful' experiences, competing as to who was in labour the longest or who had the most stitches. It's almost seen as a badge of honour to have endured something so horrific.

If, at a gathering of women, one boldly states how much she enjoyed her pregnancy and relished giving birth, she is often thought of as being smug, showing off or just not telling the truth. I've been saddened over the years by how often women have shared with me their reticence to talk about how much they enjoyed their baby's birth, how it empowered them and how they found a strength and depth of joy they hadn't known existed, for fear of upsetting others. It means that all too often pregnant women are only hearing one kind of story.

Then there's the birthing environment. Most people immediately assume they'll go to hospital to give birth.

Hospital is a place that we associate with disease and damage, where we go to be healed or repaired. Labour wards are filled with doctors and equipment that is assumed to be required. Antenatal leaflets and classes focus on pain-relief methods, describing them much in the way a restaurant menu offers you a choice of aperitif, starter and entrée: 'We'll start you off with some gas and air, then move onto diamorphine and as a main course we have an epidural on offer.' The underlying assumption, naturally, is that you will need it. If you read medical texts, brochures and websites there's little about the thoughts of women during birth. Without consciousness or volition it's almost as if the woman becomes a machine, her uterus painfully contracting, stages of labour following each other while she endures the mechanism of the child being expressed by the contortions of the uterus and birth canal. So we learn that childbirth is an ordeal, essentially painful, dangerous and something to be endured and then forgotten.

The problem is that these fears have around nine months to build. Also our brains preferentially scan for, register, store and recall unpleasant experiences. Rick Hanson, neuropsychologist and author of *Buddha Brain: the practical neuroscience of happiness, love and wisdom*, says our brain is like Velcro for bad experiences and stories and Teflon for the good. Think about it: if you go to a good restaurant you may tell a handful of friends; if you go to a bad one you tell twenty. You may even write a scathing review online and tell thousands! The negative stays with us far longer than the positive, so any positive stories you may hear of childbirth are drowned out by the unrealistic TV portrayals and the images you've been given by others.

Television *could* be an incredibly valuable way of decreasing fear of birth. Once or twice in a series of *One Born Every Minute* there is a calm birth, often in water and darkness, and, although there's a tendency for it to be shouted down by the dramatic births shown either side of it, for some viewers it can act as a beacon of hope. A few years ago there was a young couple shown: they were excited and optimistic and had no fearful or negative expectations of birth. She gave birth in water with headphones on and her partner nearby stroking her. For about two years I had women coming to my classes saying 'I want to be like the lady in the red bikini!'

If the normalcy of birth were deemed interesting enough to be on television regularly, I truly believe the fear that surrounds it would dramatically reduce.

How does fear impact birth?

We've seen how powerfully hormones operate during the birth process, with humans and indeed all female mammals releasing those helpful birth hormones, oxytocin and endorphins, when undisturbed. This allows birth to start and progress well. So what gets in the way? The short answer is fear.

To understand why, we need to take a quick look at our autonomic nervous system (ANS). The ANS operates mostly below the level of consciousness, constantly responding to our environment and thoughts to regulate many bodily systems and their responses to changing conditions.

The ANS has two subsystems – the sympathetic (SNS) and the parasympathetic (PNS) nervous systems. While both are always present, one is more dominant than the other depending on what's happening around and within us. Parasympathetic activation is the normal resting state of your body, brain and mind. It's variously referred to as the calm, confident or relaxation response. When the PNS is in charge our body is regulating itself, conserving energy: it is responsible for the ongoing, steady state of affairs. The more deeply relaxed you are, the more your body brings itself into a state of balance.

The SNS, by contrast, is stimulated when we feel threatened or challenged. It is the body's defence mechanism, often referred to as the 'freeze, flight or fight' response. Intended as a short-term protection mechanism, this stress response causes our body to speed up our heart rate, increase our blood sugar, suppress our immune system, reduce insulin production, pump out stress hormones such as adrenaline and cortisol and reduce the blood supply to our digestive organs. This increase in heart rate and blood pressure sends blood to the main limbs of the body: the legs so you can run away from the threat, the arms so you can fight it and the neo-cortex of the brain, the more modern 'thinking brain', so that you can figure out what to do to save yourself. Non-emergency systems in the body shut down to save energy, so digestion and reproduction systems will slow down and halt. You don't have time to sit and have a meal or make love when dealing with an emergency!

Although few people reading this face daily threats to their bodily existence, many live in a prolonged state of fight or flight, generating stress in response to bad traffic, disagreements, or in pregnancy continued images and stories of horrific childbirth. You'll recognise certain symptoms whenever you've felt stressed or anxious: heart palpitations, feeling nauseous, unable to eat or think clearly, feeling jittery and shaky. Because the subconscious mind doesn't know the difference between real and imagined events it will create physical changes within your body when it is faced with danger, whether that danger is perceived or real. Think about the last time you watched a frightening film and any physical reactions you might have had, despite the fact it wasn't real or happening to you! Many of my CBT clients are seeking help for physical problems such as IBS, colitis, insomnia, headaches – all caused by overstimulating the sympathetic system and flooding the body with adrenaline time and time again. The natural balance of the body is interrupted over and over and physical symptoms produced by anxiety and fear are debilitating to our health and well-being.

The two wings of the ANS are connected like a see-saw: when one goes up, the other goes down. They cannot coexist, so adrenaline will halt the production of oxytocin and endorphins. Thus the effect of fear on the birth process becomes very clear.

A woman who is frightened, stressed or feels threatened in any way will produce stress hormones. Three things you do not need to give birth are your legs, your arms or your 'thinking brain', but that's where the oxygenated blood is now sent to deal with the perceived threat. All of that oxygenated blood is being diverted away from the one place we need it most – the muscles of the uterus – so now they become resistant and tight. Rather than working together they're effectively pulling against each other, causing pain. The muscles of the cervix are no longer soft and pliable, so, rather than thinning and opening, the cervix remains tightly closed and the baby is pushing down on a tight band of muscle. The clinical term for this has become known as 'failure to progress' during labour. If a woman hears that phrase during her baby's birth, who does she think is failing? She believes her body cannot birth. Is that going to help her relax or is she going to be more stressed? She feels uncomfortable, is told that 'nothing's happening', and so she becomes anxious and stressed for herself and her baby, thereby producing more adrenaline… and so it continues.

A woman who is free from fear, and feels safe and unobserved, will produce oxytocin and endorphins freely and her body will follow the design we admired in Chapter 2. The cooling, steadying influence of the PNS helps you think clearly, quiets the mind and allows the helpful hormones of birth to flow freely.

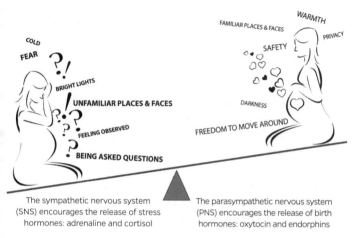

How the autonomic nervous system (ANS) affects birth.

The sympathetic nervous system (SNS) encourages the release of stress hormones: adrenaline and cortisol

The parasympathetic nervous system (PNS) encourages the release of birth hormones: oxytocin and endorphins

Oxytocin triggers the muscles to work together in surges, and these surges stimulate more oxytocin and endorphins, which produce more surges in a positive feedback loop.

Anything that disturbs a labouring woman's sense of safety and privacy will disrupt the birth process. Unfortunately, most of modern obstetrics involves disturbance, observation and monitoring, internal examinations, brightly-lit rooms, people coming and going and clock watching (implying there is a safe time frame) – all these inhibit a birthing woman, just as they would any other mammal.

The illustration above demonstrates how the nervous system affects birth and the circumstances that can encourage the flow of helpful and unhelpful hormones during birth.

Is there really such a thing as pain-free birth?

Undisturbed birth does not imply that birth will be pain free. The stress hormones released in birth are equivalent to

those of an endurance athlete, which reflects the magnitude of this event, and explains some of the sensations of birth. And like a marathon runner, a woman's task in birth is not to avoid the pain – which usually makes it worse – but to realise that birth is a peak bodily performance, for which our bodies are superbly designed. Dr Sarah Buckley

It stands to reason that if birth were intrinsically painful, if it were just a law of the universe, then it would be so for everyone. It isn't. HypnoBirthing mothers give testimonials of two-hour, painless labours. Home birth mothers often experience labour and birth as comfortable, or at least manageable. There are even some women who talk about orgasmic birth!

I can HONESTLY say it was PAINLESS – it was bloody exhausting but IT DID NOT HURT… it's an intense and wonderfully surreal experience and I find it hard to recall in great detail. But it really did not hurt. Lizzie

'The most important contributing cause of pain in otherwise normal labour is fear,' wrote Dr Grantly Dick-Read. He quotes one of the great pioneer neurologists, Sir Henry Head, who said, 'The mental state of the patient has a notoriously profound influence over the pains originating in the pelvic viscera'. In other words, the interpretation of sensations arising from the uterus and birth path may be influenced in the most astonishing of ways by the thoughts and expectations of the woman concerned.

A woman about to start her first labour has been told to expect certain sensations. If she has read books and attended HypnoBirthing classes she will be well aware of all the hormones at play in her body, how they're designed to allow her muscles to soften and open and what she can do to help that process. She has surrounded herself with a support team and feels safe, even though there may be a sense of nervous anticipation. The tightening and release of the uterine muscles will be a new experience to her, although she may have recognised them warming up in recent days and weeks and practised her breathing and movements to see how her body responds to it. She has learnt how those muscles work together and can almost see it in her mind; she knows it's productive and progressive, every surge bringing her baby closer to her. She is calm and excited.

On the other hand, if her preparation has involved watching dramatic TV programmes, hearing horror stories of how 'childbirth is the most painful thing you'll ever go through', 'it's like having every single bone in your body broken', or 'it's like being murdered' (these are actual phrases some of my mums have been told when pregnant), then her interpretation of these sensations will almost certainly be pain. The body immediately flies into protective gear and activates the freeze, flight or fight response, producing adrenaline, draining blood from the uterus, tightening muscles, creating resistance and… whaddaya know, bam! She feels pain. As you go through life, your brain acquires expectations based on your experiences and messages received, particularly negative ones. If it expects pain, or even just the threat of it, it pulses fear signals. If we *expect* pain, and are focused on it, we are likely to experience it, even when it's not there.

Some hypnobirthing models don't mention the word pain, as the mere suggestion of it creates an expectation of it. The trouble with the word pain is that it has a completely subjective meaning for each and every one of us. The most widely used definition states: 'Pain is an unpleasant sensory and emotional experience associated with actual or potential tissue damage'. The biological purpose of pain interpretation is protective. It tells us something is wrong, that we should remove our hand from that hot stove, or seek help for a broken or fractured limb. As Dick-Read pointed out 'There is no physiological function in the body which gives rise to pain in the normal course of health.' In a normal, unmedicated birth, the pain of labour isn't pathologic. It's actually productive, signalling your body how much oxytocin and endorphins to make, indicating when your body needs you to push and when something is wrong. There are known variables that contribute to pain in labour, including positioning (of both mother and baby), tension, environmental factors, obstetric management and a multitude of other things under the control of the mother. Could it be that a mother's choices, in pregnancy and during the labour and birth, have an impact on her experience? Absolutely.

Labour surges come in waves, building gradually. There is a rhythm to the hormones being released in pulsations and the muscles join in this rhythm. Though you may not have control over these surges – it's an involuntary action after all – you do have control over how you respond to them. It can be a powerful and intense sensation; these sensations have a role and help guide how a woman moves during labour to help her baby be born. These women are aware of the intensity and power of birth, but they don't call it pain. I've heard them say it's the most intense experience of their life, I've heard them describe it as 'surreal' and 'unlike anything else I've ever experienced'. By being more descriptive and open to it you can change the experience and take that power back to yourself, rather than it being something done to you. Once you understand how those muscles function, and can visualise what's happening as you feel them working, it changes how you feel about it. It feels achievable, it feels progressive, it feels right. It can't be bigger than you, because it is you. Birthing is powerful, and so are you.

There is a secret in our culture, and it's not that birth is painful. It's that women are strong. Laura Stavoe Harm

Now that you understand the theory of the fear-tension-pain cycle you may think, 'OK, I get it. I know how my body works and that will be enough'. However, simply consciously knowing something does not give us control over it.

Dr Amali Lokugamage is a consultant obstetrician and gynaecologist in London. Her experience of home birth led to her book *The Heart in the Womb*, in which she acknowledges:

> *Throwing facts and figures at women undoubtedly helps them to understand their choices, but it is more important that women are guided to unlock confidence in their bodies to embrace the process of birth. Without this, an almost virulent form of fear can sabotage their innate capabilities to birth well, quite aside from any genuine medical issues. The media is rife with pregnancy disaster stories – which sell more papers – and doctors operate from the perspective of 'worst case scenarios', because the majority of their work dwells on fixing problems in pregnancy. It is up to the midwives, doulas and natural-birth experts to provide an encouraging view of normal childbirth that affirms women's basic programmed potential to give birth. When a supportive network surrounds a woman, she has more opportunity to unlock her own innate birthing wisdom.*

This is where using hypnosis for birth preparation begins, and why hypnobirthing is so very different to other forms of antenatal preparation. Rationalising fear does not prevent it. We need to attack these deep-seated beliefs and fears on a subconscious level – in other words, we need to de-hypnotise ourselves. This is what I call moving understanding from the head to the heart, and that is accomplished with hypnosis.

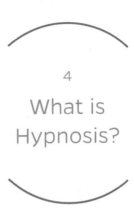

4

What is Hypnosis?

Hypnosis is as old as the human race. The phenomenon known as hypnosis has existed since the beginning of recorded history, as found in the folklore of ancient cultures and various Oriental meditation techniques. Hypnotism as a tool for health seems to have originated with the Hindus of ancient India, who often took their sick to 'sleep temples' to be cured by hypnotic suggestion, as in ancient Egypt and Greece. Despite recent decades of scientific research into the benefits of hypnosis, it's surprising how it continues to be misunderstood and judged negatively on the basis of misinformation and simple prejudice. People often react negatively to the *word* hypnosis but virtually never react negatively to the description of the *process* of hypnosis.

Hypnosis is a state of inner absorption, concentration and focused attention. It is like using a magnifying glass to focus the rays of the sun and make them more powerful. Similarly, when our minds are concentrated and focused, we are able to use our minds more powerfully.

Everyone has experienced a trance state many times, but we don't usually call it hypnosis. All of us have been so absorbed in thought – while reading a book, driving or on the bus to work – that we fail to notice what is happening around us. Conversely we can be so 'in the zone' – a pianist performing a complicated piece of music, or an athlete tuning out a crowd to focus on their best performance – that we are not conscious. While we were 'zoned out', or 'in the zone', another level of consciousness, which we refer to as our unconscious mind, took over. These are very focused states of attention, similar to hypnosis.

Once couples have heard the rationale behind using hypnosis in preparation for and during childbirth, it makes sense. But first we must deal with the common misunderstandings about hypnosis.

Who's in control?

Hypnosis isn't something someone does to you. Don't expect to be greeted by swinging pendulums or chants of 'look into my eyes' when you first attend a hypnobirthing class. Stage hypnosis has done much to devalue the therapeutic value of hypnosis and has led to the mistaken belief that the hypnotic state is brought about by someone else, who can then control your actions.

Anyone can and does access the hypnotic state several times a day. We are always aware and in control during hypnosis. When 'zoning out', reading a book or daydreaming on the bus, if something or someone demanded our attention we could deal with it, but we could also choose to ignore it and stay nice and relaxed.

Think about when you are watching a film. You switch off your critical 'thinking' brain and sink into a relaxed, very focused state in which you suspend disbelief and become absorbed in the story and characters. This too is the hypnotic state. In fact, what makes watching films and reading books so enjoyable is that we let ourselves believe that we are there in the story or in the film, rather than in our real lives (where we may have anxieties or a list of things to do) – we hypnotise ourselves.

In this sense, all hypnosis is self-hypnosis. It's something we do for ourselves. When someone works with a hypnotherapist or listens to a hypnosis recording they are allowing the hypnotherapist to guide them on a journey. A trained therapist will have a good idea of what your goal is and a good idea of how best to guide you there, but it is up to you whether you choose to go on that journey, much in the same way as you might choose to 'get into' a good book or film.

A hypnotherapist can suggest that you close your eyes, they can suggest that you focus your attention on something or imagine a scene or feeling, but they certainly can't make you do any of those things. Far from causing you to be out of control, hypnosis allows you to use more of your potential. Learning self-hypnosis is the ultimate act of self-control.

Unconscious thinking

While in this altered state of consciousness, the unconscious is more open to us. The unconscious part of our mind stores all the messages we've received in life, and from the imprints held there we formulate emotions, beliefs and thoughts. You could think of your unconscious brain as like the biggest computer hard drive in the world. It stores everything you've ever read, seen, heard and thought, filed away until you need that information.

So everything you've ever read, seen, heard and thought about childbirth is stored there, all those unfiltered, unchallenged messages from the television, films, newspapers, friends and family. It's not given much thought until you become pregnant and at some point look to see what you know and understand about giving birth, only to be confronted by these messages. If only negative images of birth are there, then who in their right mind would be looking forward to that? It's actually rational that you'd be fearful of such an experience. This is where hypnosis for birth preparation steps in.

When in the hypnotic state, the conscious mind – the part of your brain that you're always aware of, the narrator in your life, constantly talking you through your day about how well (or not) you're doing, reminding you of all that you have to do, wondering about the future, ruminating on the past – is occupied, so we can bypass it and feed more beneficial messages into the unconscious. Replacing those images and thoughts of what birth is with more helpful, not to mention truthful, images means that your starting point, your belief system, is now changed. Rather than being anxious and fearful, instead you are calm and confident. A little apprehensive, naturally, but more excited and prepared.

Brain training

There is much we can do to help train the brain before and during childbirth. In preparation for birth we use hypnosis to help counter-balance all the messages we've been fed about the horrors of childbirth and build on the intuitive trust and confidence a woman can have in her body's ability to birth.

I've mentioned already that because of how our brains have evolved, we have what's called 'the negativity bias' to remember and experience negative experiences more than positive ones. It is well documented. The short story is that tens of thousands of years ago, if we were foraging for food, but paid attention and remembered scenarios that posed a threat to survival, we lived to eat the next day. We might have a bad day where the threats were pretty constant, we might not have had much for dinner that night, but we lived to eat the next day. If we didn't pay close attention to threats, a meagre dinner would be the least of our worries. Now you are the culmination of all your ancestors, and they were the ones who were *really* good at the fight or flight response, because they looked out for potential threats and survived to reproduce. All this means that we are 'hardwired' toward these tendencies. This is why we remember the more dramatic birth stories we've been told, and why the screamy births stay with us more than the quieter, calmer ones.

The good news is that there's something we can do about it.

Modern neuroscientific research is now telling us that the brain is not really 'hardwired': it continues to create new neural pathways and alter existing ones in order to adapt to new experiences, learn new information and create new memories. Every time we think a specific thought, a specific pathway of neurons fires up, neurotransmitters are released and synapses are subtly altered. With repetition, this pathway is strengthened. There is an oft-used expression: 'neurons that fire together, wire together'. When pleasure chemicals such as oxytocin and endorphins are produced they strengthen the neural circuits that are active, making them more likely to fire together in the future. Our brain's structure is a culmination of all the thoughts and experiences we have had up to this very moment. So repeated practice of self-hypnosis, which encourages production of pleasure chemicals, is training and shaping your brain and mind, increasing what's positive and decreasing what's negative. Practices such as mindfulness meditation, hypnotherapy, cognitive behavioural therapy and more, have been proven to create changes in both brain structure and the experience of the person doing the practice. It's known as neuroplasticity and it tells us that we do not have to be victims of our current brain structure/programming/

conditioning. We have a choice! We can choose to think differently, feel differently, experience life differently.

This is the reason why hypnosis is so powerful and can be so beneficial. Hypnosis gives direct access to our subconscious mind, which can accept suggestions literally without the critical factor of the conscious mind. We can then speed up the process of rewiring our nerve cells, to speed up positive changes in our lives.

While a lot of the 'work' of hypnobirthing is done before birth, in training our brain to think positively about birth and our abilities, we use the hypnotic state to help during the birth process too. There has been much written about the function of the human brain in labour and birth, in particular the distinction between the neo-cortex – the newer, rational part of the brain, the thinking brain – and the primal brain, which governs instinct. It is the primal brain which secretes all the hormones necessary for childbirth, while stimulation of the neo-cortex can actually interfere by inhibiting that hormone release. This is why Michel Odent, the French obstetrician with a steadfast commitment to celebrating a woman's innate birthing brilliance, is often quoted as saying 'Never disturb the neo-cortex of a labouring woman!'

Helping a woman give birth means helping her reduce the activity in the rational brain. By better understanding how the brain works and changes – how it gets emotionally hijacked or settles into calmness, how it makes harmful choices or wise ones – you can take more control of your brain and therefore your mind. And since your nervous system is controlled by your unconscious mind, controlling your mind allows greater control of your nervous system. Practising self-hypnosis is to practise stepping away from the neo-cortex and becoming more familiar and comfortable with the primal brain, or what Ina May Gaskin calls the monkey self: 'Remember your monkey self knows how to do this really well. Your brain isn't very reliable as a guide of how to be during childbirth, but your monkey self is.'

It's not all in the mind

Aside from giving us the chance to address our beliefs and expectations, the hypnotic state has tremendous health benefits. The less aware you are of what's going on in your body, the more it just 'does its thing' unchecked. If you can regulate and be tuned in to your body's reactions, you stand a far better chance of making mindful, healthier and more helpful choices.

In hypnosis, your body releases stress and reverses the effects of the flight-or-fight response.

The emotional effects of sitting quietly and going within are profound. The deep state of rest produced by hypnosis triggers the brain to release neurotransmitters, including dopamine, serotonin, oxytocin, and endorphins. Each of these naturally occurring brain chemicals has been linked to different aspects of relaxation and happiness.

- Oxytocin (the same chemical whose levels rise during sexual arousal and breastfeeding) is a pleasure hormone. It creates feelings of calm, contentment and security, while reducing fear and anxiety. It is the hormone that kick-starts labour and is produced in abundance when you meet your baby for the first time, to enhance bonding and attachment.
- Endorphins are most commonly known as the chemicals that create the exhilaration during exercise. These neurotransmitters play many roles related to wellbeing, including decreased feelings of pain and stress reduction. They help keep muscles soft and pliable and so work in the way in which they're designed, effortlessly and comfortably.

- Dopamine plays a key role in the brain's ability to experience pleasure, feel rewarded, and maintain focus.
- Serotonin has a calming effect. It eases tension and helps us feel less stressed and more relaxed and focused. Low levels of this neurotransmitter have been linked to migraines, anxiety, bipolar disorder, apathy, feelings of worthlessness, fatigue, and insomnia.

You'll now also recognise the important role these hormones play during childbirth. It's no coincidence that the same hormones are produced during hypnosis as during an undisturbed birth. The conditions conducive to releasing these hormones are the very same ones that help switch off the neo-cortex and allow us to tune into our primal instinct.

Can everyone be hypnotised?

When I first introduce clients to hypnosis, they often ask 'Is this what I'm supposed to experience?' or 'Am I doing it right?' The assumption is that there has to be more, something profound and deeply moving. An awareness of breathing and narrowing one's focus of attention doesn't strike people as profound or mysterious enough to justify what they may have heard about the 'amazing' experiences of friends and colleagues who may have recommended using hypnosis to them.

Sometimes clients will go into a much lighter hypnotic state and, although this is more unusual, they will tell me that they hear everything, may not feel particularly relaxed and start to wonder if it's really working. Others find it easier to drift off and in fact have no recollection of what's been said during hypnosis and so worry that they were asleep and missed out on it all. Your experience with hypnosis will be unique to you and you may find that it changes over time and with practice. Most commonly people feel themselves drift in

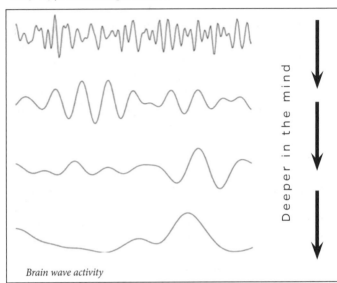

Brain wave activity

and out of lighter and deeper awareness.

Our brain functions on a small amount of electricity, much like a computer. This electrical current vibrates and pulses at various speeds. The brainwave spectrum divides into bands with different associated states.

In the last seventy years, daily human life has created a new atmosphere of beta waves in the world through modern technology; we are being agitated by beta, which in turn has created an epidemic of insomnia, digestive and other stress-related disorders. We therefore benefit from techniques to get out of beta and into alpha brainwave patterns. Research has shown many benefits of 'going to the alpha and theta levels', and these are the states associated with hypnosis. The feeling of drifting between lighter and deeper relaxation, hearing some of what's being said and then missing a bit, is this dance between alpha and theta. It's natural and it's beneficial to your health.

Beta
Normal waking state of consciousness. You are in beta reading this book. Higher levels are associated with anxiety and flight or fight response.

Alpha
Relaxed focus, day-dreaming, pre-sleep/pre-waking, drowsiness, meditation, well of creativity, awareness expands and fears vanish. Beginning of access to unconscious mind.

Theta
Deep relaxation, dreaming sleep. Insight, intuition and inspiration found here. Emotional tensions are released, which is important for well-being.

Delta
Unconscious, dreamless sleep. Certain frequencies in the delta range also trigger the release of human growth hormones, so it is beneficial for healing and regeneration.

Associated mental activity

So you can relax and let go of any preconceptions around deep or light hypnosis states. I frequently have people in my practice who claim they were never in hypnosis but still make profound changes. Depth of trance state is not an indicator of whether it's working.

If you've had experience of meditation, guided visualisations with yoga or therapy, you can bring the benefit of all your experience to your hypnobirthing preparation. If you haven't had these experiences then think about whether you've ever daydreamed, if you've ever caught yourself 'waking up' after drifting off while walking, cycling or driving, or whether you have experienced that world of 'in between' when first waking up in the morning or just before dropping off to sleep. If you have then you have already experienced the hypnotic state, and it's this natural state that you'll use with hypnobirthing.

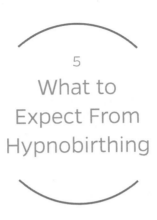

5
What to Expect From Hypnobirthing

Women have, of course, been giving birth for hundreds of thousands of years. Women's bodies are designed perfectly to birth their babies naturally. The statistical facts are that the majority of women can and do birth naturally. This is where hypnobirthing books and classes begin.

You will learn the physiological aspects of the birthing body, how the uterine muscles work and the cocktail of hormones that help. You will fully understand how all the birthing mother's muscles work in harmony, and are able to do this most efficiently if she is as relaxed as possible; and how a relaxed body is achieved by having a relaxed and confident mind. In hypnobirthing, women are taught a range of techniques to achieve a deep state of relaxation during pregnancy, labour and birth. These are hugely beneficial to both mother and baby. The methods taught include specific breathing techniques, visualisations, mindfulness, massage and self-hypnosis. Together these techniques give the body the best possible chance to do as nature intended. Learning about how the birthing body works fills a woman with trust and confidence that she can give birth naturally, and the techniques taught give her the tools to do so.

Hypnobirthing includes a lot of seemingly little things that come together to create a powerful shift in the way you're thinking and feeling about childbirth. There isn't one technique or tool that acts as a magic wand to remove fear and anxiety; instead using a wide range of techniques, both on a conscious and unconscious level, allows this subtle, yet very powerful process to occur.

When do I start hypnobirthing?

The general rule of thumb is sooner rather than later. This kind of brain training can take some time, particularly when there are deep-seated fears. Hypnobirthing teaches a mother and her partner how to relax and enjoy the pregnancy more too, so of course it makes sense to start earlier to gain the maximum benefit.

That said, one of the most dramatic turn-arounds I've seen happened for a mother who came to me 37 weeks into her second pregnancy. She was traumatised by her first birth experience to the extent that she'd avoided any thought or preparation now that she was pregnant again. She came to me very open about the fact that she'd heard that hypnobirthing could help keep you calm, and all she wanted was something to help keep her calm for long enough to get to the hospital and have an epidural.

Three weeks later she birthed her son at home with just her husband and mother around her and her eldest son tucked up in bed. When we met up, months later, she said:

You wouldn't believe as an intelligent human being that you could be so easily conditioned but I heard it, it clicked, it worked.

It's breaking away from fear, breaking the cycle and letting this happen, just not interfering, just observing your body, this is you having the baby, this is you just watching it happen. Embracing every surge, each one bringing your baby closer to you and so I was waiting for them and looking forward to them so when they came I could do what I'm supposed to do with them.

I think that so many women are having babies without knowing that this is the most cherished moment in a woman's life. The most incredible moment. There are no other moments like that. It's like everything together, like the best day in your life emotionally, the best orgasm, all of the best emotional things that have happened to you all your life all in one moment together. The essence of creating a human being in one moment. It's everything that we are about. Maya

Many teachers will recommend that you wait until after your 20-week scan to join classes. I've taught some women this early who then said they would have preferred to do it later, and I've taught many, many women who wished they'd known about and engaged with hypnobirthing earlier than they did.

It's incredible, for instance, the number of women who are frightened by the threat of a c-section because of a low-lying placenta at the 20-week scan. It's important to know that the vast majority of women who have a low-lying placenta in the middle of pregnancy will not be affected in the later weeks. As the uterus expands the placenta is moved away from the cervix so that at the end of pregnancy only a tiny percentage of women have the condition of true placenta praevia (where the placenta is covering the cervix). The whole situation causes unnecessary stress to women who could be happily enjoying their pregnancy and preparing for birth. If the placenta truly covers the cervix by the time a baby is ready to be born then a c-section is necessary and we can be grateful that such help is available. HypnoBirthing helps prepare couples for a caesarean birth as well as a 'normal' birth.

The one thing I'd like to get across is that hypnobirthing is for *everyone*. Whether you're convinced you're going to want an epidural or know you're considered 'high risk', it helps everyone, in all circumstances.

Can I teach myself hypnobirthing?

The short answer is yes. It is possible to read a book and listen to hypnosis recordings on your own if there isn't a teacher nearby or you can't afford a course. Many teachers offer concessionary places, so it's always worth asking and there are some who offer Skype sessions and home study programmes. There have been no studies exploring the difference in effectiveness between self-taught and professionally taught courses; it's easy to appreciate, however, that working with a teacher will provide much more information and a tailored approach to your specific fears and concerns that you couldn't get from a book alone.

There is so much more to a hypnobirthing course than just following a book, so here are some tips to get the most out of hypnobirthing if you're not able to join a class.

Top tips for doing it yourself

- Just reading about hypnobirthing is not enough. Self-hypnosis is a skill that needs to be learnt and effectiveness increases with repeated practice. You can't read a book about how to play a musical instrument and then assume you can play it. Insight and proficiency come about through practice, and research shows that when you read about a subject you retain about 10 per cent of the information, but when you actively practise you retain about 90 per cent!

- It's often wrongly thought that HypnoBirthing is just relaxation classes... Given the negativity bias of the brain it takes an active effort to internalise positive experience and expectation. Conditioning the mind and body takes time, and repeated practice in all areas is key. Stop watching adrenaline-fuelled births on television and seek out inspiring births on YouTube, mybirth.tv and hypnobirthing websites. Choose the books you read with care (there's suggested reading at the back of this book) and surround yourself with positive affirmations and people.

- Get your partner involved: it's important they read the same things as you and experience the recordings too; there's a lot of discipline required to do this by yourselves. Many couples appreciate classes as it's dedicated time to focus on this baby and pregnancy. You won't *find* the time to do hypnobirthing, you have to make the time to focus on it.

- Join a positive birth group. If you can't afford classes during your pregnancy, joining a free positive birth group is a wonderful opportunity to meet other expectant parents who are looking to prepare for and experience birth positively. Check out the Positive Birth Movement, a grassroots movement with hundreds of groups around the world. positivebirthmovement.org

- Plug in online: there is a general hypnobirthing page on Facebook, which is an open forum you can join to ask questions of other parents, and there are plenty of hypnobirthing teachers on there too. Most hypnobirthing teachers have valuable resources freely available on their websites too, so make the web work for you.

Working with a teacher

Unlike other antenatal courses where you simply book a date rather than a teacher, with hypnobirthing you can choose who to work with. While most 'methods' have a syllabus, every teacher will bring their own skills and life experience and what they bring to the course can often be as important as the type of course they offer.

As with any kind of service you'd do well to do a little research into what's available locally to you. If you're looking for a plumber, a hairdresser, a doctor or a therapist you'll ask friends for recommendations, so ask around and do an internet search. Are there any teachers in your area? What is their background? Are they qualified hypnotherapists or professional birth workers? Do they have other skills and experience that you feel is important? Do your homework and always check that a teacher is qualified and certified. Hypnobirthing is not, as yet, formally regulated and therefore anyone who teaches in the field of antenatal education could make reference to hypnobirthing in their material. It's your responsibility to seek out someone who has undergone thorough, officially recognised training to ensure you get the best help.

It's an old adage but it's true that you often get what you pay for. Independent childbirth educators are specialists in what they do. We do it because we're passionate about giving mothers to be and their partners confidence and choice. We will give you independent, up-to-date, evidence-based information, rather than hospital policy, and as this is our way of making a living it is important to us that the course is worth it to you. We depend on good word of mouth and most of the couples I teach come through personal recommendation because friends and colleagues have left the course feeling calm, confident, empowered and excited, and they know they have my support right up to and beyond the day their baby arrives.

Hypnobirthing can be taught in group or private classes. Some teachers offer weekly sessions, others full days. Again there are no studies to show if there's a difference in effectiveness and, when asked, a couple will often favour the method they chose for themselves. There's much to recommend joining other local pregnant couples in a group course. It's instinctive for pregnant women to want to meet with others and share the experience and this has been shown to be hugely beneficial for all. Questions may come up in a group environment that you hadn't thought to ask and are grateful someone else did. Lifetime friends are often made in antenatal courses, and with hypnobirthing you can be assured that the others there are likely to have a similar outlook on life to you.

> *The sessions built on ideas from the book as well as including clips from inspirational documentaries about natural childbirth. We were led through a number of guided hypnotic techniques; one of my husband's favourite aspects of the course! Through experiencing the effects themselves, our partners were able to support us all the more in our practice and of course ultimately during labour. We had lots of discussion time which enabled us to get to know the other couples and share thoughts and ideas; through hearing about my homebirth plans and seeing videos of homebirths on the course, two out of the three other women went on to book with the homebirth team and successfully achieve them! Incidentally, we have kept in touch with these couples and have become good friends.* Carly

Self-hypnosis is practised as a solo exercise and clinical hypnosis is typically structured as a guided experience. A clinical hypnotherapist will recognise and respond to the unique attributes of the client in front of them and tailor the approach accordingly. For those who cannot make, or prefer not to attend, group classes, private sessions mean that a teacher, particularly a trained hypnotherapist, can adapt and tailor hypnosis sessions for those they are working with.

A hypnobirthing teacher in your area will also know your local hospitals and midwives; the birthing world is often a very close-knit community, and hypnobirthing teachers will have first-hand recommendations and help plug you into your local support network of therapists and support groups so you feel fully supported through your pregnancy, birth and beyond.

So what will you actually DO in hypnobirthing?

Watch your language

> *Words are more powerful than drugs.*
> Rudyard Kipling

How we talk about birth affects how we're thinking about it. How we think about birth affects how we're feeling towards it. How we feel affects how we behave. The language of childbirth has become very medical, and as a result can be either confusing or downright scary. In HypnoBirthing we tend to use a much softer, more descriptive language – in most programmes we don't experience contractions, but surges. The word 'contraction' is rather a harsh, mechanical word that creates a sense of tightening; the uterine muscles do indeed tighten during a 'surge', but they also release and HypnoBirthing couples focus on releasing and relaxing. The word surge reminds us that it is something which builds and then subsides, rather than just tenses and tightens. Mothers experience a 'birth show' instead of a 'bloody show', they become aware of 'warm-ups' rather than 'Braxton Hicks', and their membranes don't 'rupture', they 'release'. Small changes can make a world of difference.

Traditional birthing programmes teach distinct stages of labour – latent labour and established labour, first stage, second stage and third stage of birth. Labour stages are merely chartable numbers developed as assessment tools for medical care providers. For the mother, birth is a continuum: when she is deeply relaxed it unfolds so that the thinning and opening of her cervix naturally progresses to the downward phase when her baby makes his way down to emerge into the world. The language used in hypnobirthing is more descriptive, easily understood and reinforces the approach that birth is a family rather than a medical event.

Affirmations

It is our thoughts about what happens that determine our experience of anything in life. What we say to ourselves about ourselves, about others, and about the events happening around us is the source of our emotions and makes up our reality on a daily basis. Becoming aware of these thoughts, working with them, and consciously choosing the subsequent mindset can drastically change our world for the better. With HypnoBirthing we recognise that we always have the choice to think positively or negatively. We learn to think, talk and feel positively about birth, which leads to an increased chance of a positive birth experience. You've already read how our brain has a bias towards the more negative in a (mostly) misguided attempt to keep us alive, and so remembers the more dramatic, unhelpful stories and thoughts about birth.

Similarly, it's always easier to think the worst about ourselves.

Years of negative or unhelpful self-talk will have an impact. If you continue to feed your mind negative self-talk, eventually you will end up developing an unhealthy belief about yourself or your abilities. This belief will in turn provoke more negative self-talk and your emotions and behaviour will be hugely influenced by it. Negative self-talk will result in a vicious cycle and a negative self-fulfilling prophecy. You might recognise negative self-talk from the following expressions: 'That sounds difficult', 'I don't think I can do it', 'I'll probably fail'. If you fill your mind with such thoughts from the moment you wake up until you go to bed, whenever you think about yourself and your abilities, their negativity will impact on you in a fundamental way.

Like everything else your self-talk is part of a process of change. First you start to think about something. Then you start to repeat it, and before long it becomes the way you think. It becomes normal and usual. If you are thinking negatively and don't stop to question the truth or helpfulness of your thoughts, and continue to repeat the same old nonsense, then it becomes a habit. Negative self-talk is nothing more than an old, bad habit, and it can be changed.

> *Even if it has not been your habit throughout your life*
> *so far, I recommend that you learn to think positively*
> *about your body.*
>
> Ina May Gaskin

Affirmations are positive statements that you say to yourself. HypnoBirthing programmes share with you suggested birthing affirmations that will build trust and confidence in nature's way of birthing. 'I trust my body and my baby', 'I am calm and confident', 'I listen to my instincts', 'My baby arrives safely in their own time': statements that reflect what you'd *like* to think then become absorbed as your new truth with repetition. Repeated practice of affirmations can take many forms. Saying them to yourself, out loud, is very powerful. Yes, it feels weird if you've not done it before, but you get over it very quickly. I'm a big fan of visual reminders so writing affirmations on post-it notes, creating beautiful postcards of images and words and putting them up around the house is great. The most common places I find them in people's homes are by the loo, on the bathroom mirror, by the bed, next to the kettle, on the fridge door – anywhere you're likely to see them repeatedly. When you see it, you read it; when you read it you're saying it to yourself. All hypnosis for birth programmes encourage this and also provide recordings in which affirmations are recited and repeated over music. Listening to a recording is a very easy way of engaging with these new beliefs. I find most women use these when commuting to work (unless they're driving), walking, swimming, taking a bath and as they go to sleep. There comes a point when you're not sure if it's an affirmation said externally or your own thoughts and this can happen quickly, within a few weeks.

In a way it is 'fake it 'til you make it', and it's important to know you don't need to *believe* the messages in the beginning. It's a phenomenon of the way our minds work – neuroplasticity working for you – that repetition means these preferred messages become absorbed as your truth.

> *Our life is what our thoughts make it.*
>
> Marcus Aurelius, 180AD

Contrary to popular opinion, affirmations are not a new idea. As emperor of Rome, Marcus Aurelius wrote a series of personal philosophies intended for himself while on campaign between 170 AD and 180 AD; these would later be published as the book

Meditations. His writing has remained relevant for almost 2,000 years because he wrote as a man, not an emperor. He wrote about his fear, his emotions, his sense of the fleetingness of life and the importance of living in and savouring the moment. The central themes of *Meditations* are repetitive. Considering that this was essentially his notebook, he was most likely engaging in behaviour modification through written affirmations. Using positive affirmations is a technique that's been around for thousands of years because it works!

Focus on what you want, rather than what you don't want

You can train and strengthen your attention just like any other mental ability and the techniques taught in hypnobirthing are doing just that. Our thoughts are made up of the stories we've been told and the images we've seen, so HypnoBirthing will encourage you to surround yourself with what you want, rather than what you don't want.

What we think will 'probably happen' in a situation sets a filter for all the information coming towards us, so what we fear often comes upon us like a self-fulfilling prophecy. The law of attraction – that what you think about you bring about – has been written about for years, and in HypnoBirthing we view birth as a family event rather than a medical one. Being mindful of the messages you're receiving from the media, from the people around you and from your own head is important. Choosing to surround yourself with positive, helpful messages is important.

Check out your belief system about birth – is it yours or someone else's? It's time to dump the negative and embrace the positive. Avoid all websites, TV shows, negative birthing stories and books that are medically orientated. Focusing on what you do want doesn't mean to the exclusion of what might happen. Hypnobirthing is not advocating anyone carelessly throw caution to the wind and totally ignore possible consequences, we just do not dwell on and feed the negative ones. We have highly skilled midwives and obstetricians to deal with the small percentage of the 'what if's' of birth, so give your thoughts and energy to the positive possibilities. It is just as easy. Aside from potentially affecting the outcome, it makes the experience of pregnancy so much more pleasant as you go through it. The power of birth comes from within and when your attention is steady, so is your mind. It is not rattled or hijacked by thoughts and feelings, but stably present and grounded.

I know that the best way to counter the effects of frightening birth stories is to hear or read inspiring ones. Though it is important to share difficult stories in order to heal, it is just as vital to tell positive stories to reduce fear, build confidence, and transmit alternative knowledge. I've been honoured to share hundreds of amazing birth stories from those I've worked with and I know how inspiring it is for parents-to-be.

Websites liketellmeagoodbirthstory.com, positivebirthmovement.org and homebirthersandhopefuls.com are filled with positive birth stories. There are many support groups growing around the UK where parents and parents-to-be are coming together to support and encourage each other in taking control of their birthing experience. Your hypnobirthing teacher will put you in touch with these groups and have many, many positive stories to share with you too.

Remember to breathe...

Just focusing on the breath can remind you that there is a reliable, life-sustaining process that you can enjoy and count on. Bringing awareness to breathing and allowing it to slow and become more even makes your heart beat more slowly and evenly. Slow deep breaths send the message from your lungs and heart that things aren't dangerous 'out there' in the world. All of this body-based information gets sent up to the primal part of the brain as a message of safety – the parasympathetic system responds and cooperates by calming things down even more deeply in the body.

You will learn specific breathing techniques to help with the surges of uterine action during birth. They will often change from the thinning and opening phase of birth to the more downward phase where a woman is taught how to breathe her baby out rather than use the forceful pushing we're used to seeing in dramatised childbirth.

Connecting with your body

Just performing a body scan, in which you are encouraged to focus on and become aware of different parts of the body in turn, can remind you that you are capable of greater physiological control than you sometimes realise and that the body can be a source of comfort and pleasure.

If you've ever caught yourself sitting at a computer with your shoulders hunched up around your ears, you know that we unconsciously hold a lot of tension in our bodies. Your body is constantly sending signals to your brain, reporting back as to whether we are safe and can relax or we need to be aware and ready to run or fight. In order to release tension we have to first become aware of it; we need to notice our shoulders are hunched up around our ears before we can drop them back into the frame of our body. With practice we can regularly release tension in the body and maintain a sense of calmness in the nervous system, even if it's not so calm around us.

You will often be guided through visualisations and hypnosis sessions by your teacher in class and through the use of audio recordings in your own time. These typically, but not always, begin with suggestions to close the eyes and focus on the breath as a means to relax and develop focus. The exercises

Quickly anchoring your emotions and body helps you interrupt the stress response and bring balance to your mind and body. Try this:

Remember the phrase 'soft jaw, soft hands' and repeat it to yourself whenever you need to. Softening the jaw and hands softens your resistance, limitations and inner tension. You can't get tense or nervous if you have a soft jaw and hands, and as soon as you repeat the words it will remind you to relax and breathe. Do this anytime, anywhere; eyes open or closed.

Sitting on the tube or bus feeling tired and stressed – soft jaw, soft hands and breathe…

Standing at the sink surrounded by dirty dishes and a screaming baby – soft jaw, soft hands and breathe…

About to go into an important meeting – soft jaw, soft hands and breathe…

Waiting for an antenatal appointment – soft jaw, soft hands and breathe...

then proceed to guide your attention in whatever direction will facilitate the goals of the session, such as: becoming aware of bodily sensations, releasing fears and concerns, connecting with your baby/intuition/partner. Following a spoken guide gives the rational mind something to focus on, which is the easiest form of meditation for those with active minds. A lot of hypnosis programmes will encourage your partner to help guide you into relaxation with the aid of scripts and music. This is a powerful way of connecting your feelings of safety, confidence and calmness with your partner's voice; this is, after all, the voice that will be with you during birth. Learning to anchor feelings of calmness and confidence to your partner's voice, their touch, certain aromas and imagery will mean you can recall those feelings by using those anchors during labour and birth.

In addition, massage techniques which are known to increase endorphin levels are taught to birth partners, enabling them to deepen and support the birthing mother's levels of relaxation, and ensuring that both parents can be more aware, calm, confident and in control, in order to have a more relaxed and enjoyable birthing experience.

The power of visualisation

Imagery is our oldest form of communication. Before we developed language we conveyed messages, thoughts and feelings visually. It's a powerful way of communicating with our unconscious in a way that words can't quite reach. As a formal technique some people worry about visualisation and their ability to 'do it'. The truth is anyone can learn to visualise. Bring to mind a friend or family member, someone you really like. Pretty easy, right? It doesn't take a lot of effort, it's something we can do very naturally but when people do it in the context of a technique a little too much effort goes into it so it feels unnatural and harder to do.

Recent studies have shown how the brain is stimulated by an imagined experience in exactly the same way as the actual experience. We know this instinctively too. If you see, or imagine, a picture of a beach, palm trees bathed in sunshine, waves gently lapping at the shore, you tend to automatically start to relax and breathe a little deeper. So we can use visualisation to help with relaxation, but we can also use it as a powerful tool to convey messages.

Hypnobirthing will introduce you to visual imagery that has been known, across the world, to help birthing for hundreds, if not thousands of years.

Releasing fear

It's important to understand that there is a difference between fear and concern. Concern is a normal part of pregnancy and birth. It is normal to be concerned for yourself and your baby. It is normal to wonder how you will cope/are coping with the enormous physiological changes and sensations in your body. It is normal to be concerned about the changes that will come when this new person enters your life. However, when this concern tips into fear and anxiety, when you're constantly thinking 'What if…?' it can sabotage your ability to do something about it.

Hypnobirthing offers a chance to open up the discussion about any fears and anxieties you're experiencing so you can explore how to alleviate them. It gives you a sense of the fears you can do something about, and those that serve no purpose other than to cause anxiety and tension. Hypnosis sessions are then able to address these concerns on a deeper level and encourage you to release them and replace them with more helpful messages.

We used a hypnotherapy technique whereby in a state of deep relaxation, we replaced any negative thoughts or fears around birthing with a positive image. I imagined myself, my husband Simon and two children all together surrounding our new baby in love and cuddles! It was such a vivid and joyful image and one that I carried with me for the rest of my pregnancy. The old fears I'd had were just not tangible to me any more. Claudia

Practice doesn't make perfect

I've made repeated mention of how practice is key to the success of hypnobirthing. Practice with hypnobirthing can be anything from a few minutes' breathing and bringing awareness to your body and letting go of tension in that moment, to spending twenty minutes doing massage or a script with your partner.

When I say 'practice' it often gets linked to the idea that 'practice makes perfect', which then feeds into the idea that hypnobirthing is teaching a woman how to give birth. If she reads enough and practises enough she will pass the test and have the 'perfect' birth. Nothing could be further from the truth. HypnoBirthing isn't teaching you how to give birth. You don't need to attend a course of any kind for that; your body and your baby already know how to bring that baby forth. What you are learning through hypnobirthing is how to gracefully step out of the way and let them get on with it. That requires a few things:

- Trust that your body and baby *can* do this.
- Confidence that you have the right people around you and you feel safe and comfortable enough to let go.
- Familiarity with that no-brain, no thinking, relaxed state that you can easily slip into and tune out distractions.

All of this requires practice. For the perfectionists among us (I include myself here) it might be more helpful to think along the lines of 'practice makes progress'.

How will I know it's working?

The process of using hypnosis for birth preparation can be misleadingly subtle. For me, HypnoBirthing is an amalgamation of lots of little things that, when brought together, create a huge shift in mindset. The subtleness of this process can mean it's not immediately apparent for those doing it and there is sometimes incredulity in those with whom I share HypnoBirthing, a sense of 'It can't possibly be as simple as me relaxing while someone talks to me?' and yet the one thing I'm sure of is that it's the small things inside your mind that will lead to big changes in your brain and your experience of living. I've seen it happen time and time again and I've experienced it myself.

Clients will often report that they couldn't maintain focus as they either fell asleep or mundane and irrelevant thoughts sidetracked them during hypnosis. It's important to know this is normal, to be expected and that regular practice will increase focus and decrease distractibility. It's also good to know that whatever the conscious mind may miss can still be absorbed and responded to meaningfully by the unconscious. The auditory system is mechanical, so if you're falling asleep when listening to hypnosis recordings you can trust that your unconscious is listening to the suggestions and making the changes that are consistent with your intentions around birth.

Similarly if you're worrying that you 'don't feel any different' or that your mind is sidetracked, let go of 'trying' to make it work, or worrying that it isn't, and just go with it. Keep practising. All repetitive hypnobirthing practice is conditioning. However you react to hypnosis, your body will be conditioning a response to the background music, the words, and the voice. It may not always be obvious that this is happening, but it is. Your muscles react positively by letting go of tension, without your conscious mind even needing to know about it.

I'm reminded of a woman who came to me for HypnoBirthing and was terrified of the prospect of giving birth. Even after our first session she emailed me and confessed that she understood the principles behind using hypnosis, and 'got' the science of the fact that her body was built to give birth, but she still couldn't shake the feeling that it 'wouldn't work' for her. Less than a month later she was calm, confident and excited about the prospect of giving birth. We met a year later and she confessed she couldn't remember having emailed me in such a panicked state. She couldn't recall what that felt like and was rather reluctant to put herself back there in order to appreciate how far she'd come.

Once we've changed our way of thinking and behaving why would we place ourselves back where we were? Often I hear back from mums and dads-to-be who say 'we actually can't believe what our attitude to birth was before – it seems so obvious now!' Similarly, it makes me smile when I receive an email from a couple saying their baby's birth was so swift they didn't have time to use the hypnobirthing, as if it were a switch they forgot to press rather than the approach and preparation that led them to be the calm, confident, empowered parents able to create the optimal conditions in which their baby was born.

Amy – a second-time mum, initially dreading giving birth again – describes using the various techniques she learned through hypnobirthing to have a wonderful home birth

The first time I gave birth was pretty average: terrifying, agonising, prolonged and druggy. I had been dreading it since I was a girl and I thought the best I could hope for was that the baby and I would survive the ordeal. (We did.) In the run-up, I had distracted myself with things like pregnancy yoga, making an iPod playlist, renting a tens machine and reading a book about a French natural birth clinic in the 1970s, where slim, hairy women swaggered about the place before squatting to release their babies painlessly. This mish-mash of activity failed to prepare me. However, despite being tweezed into the world with forceps as I lay there numb from the waist down, Sam thrived from the minute he was born (although it took his mother a while to recover).

Early in my second pregnancy, the placenta was low so there was a chance that I'd need a planned c-section. I hardly relished this prospect, although the possibility of having labour taken out of my hands felt like a relief. When a smiling midwife later gave me the green light for a normal delivery, my heart sank and I knew I had to deal with my fear.

I didn't know whether hypnobirthing would work for me, but I certainly couldn't find evidence of anyone having regretted trying it, so I signed up for a course. It turned out that most of the reasoning behind the hypnobirthing process made sense to me. My teacher was relaxed and realistic and not at all preachy and when she talked about the 'cascade of intervention' that is so common with hospital births, she could have been describing my son's.

Simple aspects of hypnobirthing helped build my confidence and positivity during my pregnancy. The picture of a head-down baby, perfectly positioned for an easy birth, on my bedside table. The time-lapse film clips of roses unfurling which I watched in my third trimester while thinking about my cervix opening. And when the Braxton Hicks contractions – or practice surges – got going, I tried out the breathing techniques while visualising my womb as ribbons, soft and pliable getting ready to work together and my cervix opening like a flower.

My partner, Matt, and I tried out some of the other visualisation and relaxation exercises together when we could find time. I started to associate Matt's voice and presence with tranquil time-outs.

By the fourth and final class, I had decided to try for

a home birth. After watching a few films of surprisingly quiet hypnobirths, I felt that I would find it easier to be at peace and surrender myself to the process at home (even with paper-thin party walls and building site outside). I went into labour on the morning of the due date, which happened to be my birthday. I was at my mother's house with Sam and I knew just what to do. I lay on my mother's bed, alone. As the gentle surges came every half hour or so, I inhaled slowly to fill my imaginary abdominal balloons, and then pictured the ribbons and flowers as I let each balloon float away. It felt lovely to snuggle in the quiet, and let it happen. After a few hours I went to the loo and had a little bloody show (this hadn't appeared until after a day of frequent jarring contractions, the first time around) and smiled to myself. It was working. I was opening.

Matt brought me home at around midday, leaving Sam with his grandmother. I got into bed and ate some pizza and fruit and had a drink before things sped up and intensified. Suddenly it was after three, and we were progressing well. The surges were much closer and stronger – this was when I needed Matt to press the small of my back. And as I was breathing, he calmly told me to give my balloons colours, which helped lift me back into relaxation and keep going.

By the time the first midwife, Beverly, arrived I was reaching my tolerance threshold. She took one look at me and said 'baby's coming'. I sucked in some gas and air and made a lumbering mad dash down the corridor to the birthing pool. The relief I felt as the water enveloped me was immense – as though I had been on fire. It was re-energising, too.

The pushing surges kicked in almost immediately. It's

different for every woman but to me it felt like a powerful internal engine had taken over. There was nothing I could do other than try to stay relaxed and let it happen.

This is where my memory becomes a little hazy, but I think there were only three or so surges before I felt the head first break through. It was so exciting to feel her starting her journey out. I gave an elated, if slightly hysterical running commentary to Matt and Beverly. When Georgia was crowning, Beverly observed that her hands were in front of her face, making the circumference of her head area even bigger to squeeze out and putting her eyes at risk, so I should slow down. I said I'd try although I wasn't sure I had any influence over this bizarre engine. Next surge, Beverly said I could catch Georgia but I didn't quite trust my grip at this point so Matt enthusiastically stepped in.

'She's big,' said Beverly, looking impressed. All 8lb 8oz (3.8kg) of Georgia came into the world at around 6pm with her sac still intact – a rare and auspicious occurrence. Georgia started breastfeeding immediately and Matt took a photo to commemorate how we, who had felt so bewildered and helpless the first time around, had managed a dream water birth. A few hours after the delivery, I had showered and Matt and I were tucked up in bed eating treats, admiring Georgia sleeping beside us in her basket. We kept saying with amazement: 'That really couldn't have gone any better'.

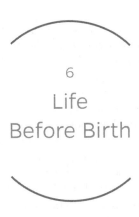

6
Life
Before Birth

I feel like I have been able to engage more and listen to my body since starting hypnobirthing, I generally feel happier and more relaxed in all aspects of life, and have even had a few lovely dreams about giving birth, which must be helpful! Most people I know seem to spend most of their pregnancy avoiding thoughts about the birth, and I think I was probably doing this before the classes. Kat

Hypnobirthing is very different from other antenatal preparation. You'll find yourself becoming aware of your emotional, mental and physical approach to giving birth: understanding how your mind and body work and how you can have more control over them is incredibly empowering and often spills into other areas of life. It will prepare you in many more ways than you first imagine.

Rather than thinking of hypnobirthing as just for birth and doing 'homework' practice, I encourage couples to use the approach and techniques to help them with everyday life. This allows it to become your unconscious, automatic approach to life. Life can be challenging; there's an unwritten law somewhere that when pregnant you should move house, renovate or at least redecorate. Bringing a child into the world throws the rest of your life into perspective and it's often a time of transition and change in more ways than one.

Learning to focus on what you want rather than what you don't want, thinking positively, calming your nervous system – all these things can help you when you're feeling anxious about a meeting or presentation at work, if there's someone annoying near you on public transport, with being nervous before an antenatal appointment, trying to stay calm when a toddler is throwing a tantrum… The skills taught in hypnobirthing are life skills, not just for birth. Indeed, integrating the approach and techniques to help you with the challenges of daily life means you're more able to reach for these tools when you need them most.

What you've given us is so much wider than the 24 (fingers crossed) hours of the birth of our kid. You've given us a mindset for life. You've educated us, which is not something either of us expected. We knew we'd learn techniques but you've opened a world up to us that will, if practised, aid our work, our home life, our time with our child way beyond the birth and our relationship. Sophie

When you're practising the hypnotic state, you're controlling your nervous system and bringing it into calmness and balance. It quietens the fight-or-flight sympathetic system since relaxed muscles send feedback to the alarm centres of the brain that all is well. You can reap the benefits of relaxation not only by initiating it in specific, stressful situations, but also by training the body 'offline' to relax automatically. Deliberately feeling safe, as you do when you practise hypnobirthing techniques, helps control that automatic tendency to look for and overreact to threats. If you know that you're naturally quite an anxious person and prone to worry, this is a wonderful opportunity to practise simple techniques to help you control your anxiety levels.

I now can't really remember how it feels to be panicky and scared about the prospect of birth and as a result have enjoyed this last stage of pregnancy more than any other time. Isobel

It's not just emotional: there can be many physical challenges a woman faces during pregnancy, mostly triggered by a combination of hormonal, physical and emotional changes taking place.

Many people, websites and books will tell you that these symptoms are a normal part of pregnancy and that you just have to 'put up with it.' However, there is considerable research which has shown that psychosocial variables have a clear influence, including levels of stress, social support and emotions relating to being pregnant. Stress in particular has been shown to increase the incidence and severity of morning sickness, insomnia and raised blood pressure due to the increase in stress hormones of adrenaline and cortisol.

So regular practice of hypnosis can have a profound effect on your health and well-being.

It's not just you...

Of course what's happening for mother is happening for baby too. Babies play a very active part in HypnoBirthing as they respond really positively to the relaxation and breathing practice, which helps baby and parents to bond before they are even born. Perinatal psychology – the study of baby and mothers' brains before and after birth – shows us that when you take time to relax and let go your baby benefits enormously. Babies in the womb respond to light, temperature, taste, vibrations, music, voices, stroking. Their brain is starting to fire and wire and they will calm and relax when you're calm and relaxed. Conversely, high levels of stress during pregnancy can fire and wire your baby's brain for over-reactivity to stress.

Author Joseph Chiltern Pearce is a well-known commentator on human intelligence, child development and subsequent adult emotional development. His interest in natural birth grew from his opinion that many child development issues stem from the neurocardiological foundations laid in fetal life, a view that led him to become a natural birth activist. He argues that a woman's pregnancy and birth should be as gentle as possible to promote the optimal natural psychobiological development of her baby. According to Chilton Pearce, if a pregnant woman is entrenched in an environment that is not wellness orientated and does not nurture her and the baby then the resulting stress chemicals will lead to emotional behaviour for survival, such as anxiety and hostility. He believes that the emotional quality of pregnancy and the birth experience can have an impact on child development.

Michel Odent has also written extensively about what he calls primal health. He says:

Primal health is built at that time when the baby is closely dependent on its mother, first in the womb, then during childbirth, and then during the period of breastfeeding. Everything that happens during this period of dependence on the mother has an influence on this basic state of health, this primal health.

Unborn babies are aware, are capable of learning and will strive to make sense of what they are feeling and experiencing. Dr Thomas Verny, in his book *The Secret Life of the Unborn Child,* describes how his interest was aroused as he noticed a pregnant friend sing a lullaby in the evenings. After the birth of her son the lullaby had a magical effect; no matter how hard he was crying that song quietened him immediately. Long before they are born, babies are thinking, feeling and even acting. They can learn and remember. I've lost count of the number of times I've been told about parents using the hypnosis recordings after a baby has been born to help calm them.

Now of course life is challenging and stressful sometimes – we can't avoid it completely. Committing to using the tools taught in hypnobirthing to help you with the stresses of daily life, and having internalised again and again a sense of calm, will mean that you are more able to face situations at work or in life in general without getting so rattled by them, without being locked into the reactive mode of the brain. You'll also know that you're helping your baby as well as yourself to cope better with what's happening for you now.

> *Megan has the same instant chill-out response to the hypnosis music that I do. I've started using it for her bedtime routine. She seems very blissed when it's on. It might be because it has that effect on me, so she calms to match my mood, but I wonder if she remembers it.*
> Kathryn

Location, location, location

So hypnobirthing practice has benefits for both parents and baby before and after birth. It helps you enjoy pregnancy and enables you to plan and prepare for your ideal birth experience. Preparation of the mind and body for any experience is essential. Does an athlete sit back in a chair and say they'll take the marathon as it comes, see how it goes? That they'll try to finish the race? Of course not. If you know you're going to face an intense physical experience you have a choice as to how you approach it. Studies have shown a relationship between childbirth outcomes and women's antenatal attitude. As you'd expect, those who are fearful report more negative birth experiences. You might be surprised to learn, however, that those with a 'take it or leave it' attitude – those who were not afraid of childbirth but appeared to have no firm attitudinal preferences concerning birth – had an increased likelihood of elective caesarean. A 2012 study conducted in Sweden and Australia said that this group of 'see how it goes' women could 'benefit from clear information regarding the potential impacts of intervention on them and their baby. They could be encouraged to take a more proactive approach to giving birth… with clear explanations and guidance from clinicians these women may be potentially positioned to avoid unnecessary intervention.'

Antenatal hypnosis is shown to increase the likelihood of normal birth and a large contributory factor in this is the confidence gained to birth in a location that is conducive to the helpful hormones of birth. Dr. Michael Rosenthal, a US obstetrician inspired by the work of Michel Odent, has famously said that, 'The first intervention in birth, that a healthy woman takes, is when she walks out the front door of her home, in labour. From that first intervention, all others will follow'.

Intuitively and anecdotally, midwives have always known that out-of-hospital birth is safe, and more satisfying for mothers, families and midwives. Because of this, midwifery innovators and leaders have striven to establish birth centres, and to promote and support home birth. The difference now is that we have strong, clear evidence to back up the knowledge. The large Birthplace study conducted in 2011 in England revealed that giving birth in a non-obstetric unit setting significantly and substantially reduces the chance of having a caesarean section, instrumental delivery or episiotomy. It concluded that women planning a home birth were more likely than women planning for birth in other settings to have a normal birth: 88 per cent of planned home births are 'normal births', compared to just under 60 per cent of planned obstetric unit births. Women giving birth in midwife-led settings, either at home or in birth centres, report feeling more satisfied with their birth experience, and that their birth positively influenced the way they felt about themselves.

Many hypnobirthing couples opt to give birth at home or in a midwife-led setting such as a birth centre; they may decide to employ a doula or independent midwives, and by creating a supportive team around them they are able to truly enjoy their pregnancy and look forward to birthing their baby.

A few weeks into the course I was a different person. This empowering feeling took hold of me and I started to see how amazing it must feel to be in control of birthing your own baby. I also began to understand the mechanics of birth much more in detail. The fear just melted away and I became more and more confident. When I went to my last midwife appointment this change must have registered with them because they offered to help me organise a home birth if I wanted to. The minute she said that I felt a wave of emotion coming up and I knew that was what I really wanted to do. Despite the last-minute change I managed to organise everything and I'm now waiting for my baby to be born in his own home. I'm aware things could always work out differently from my plans but I'm not scared any more and full of positive energy. Manuela

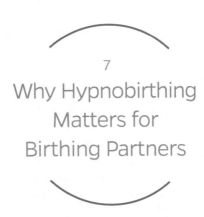

7

Why Hypnobirthing Matters for Birthing Partners

Not too long ago the perceived role of the father at his child's birth was to pace the hallways of the hospital, cigar in hand, ready to raise a glass and toast his baby's birth. These days dads are often expected to be at the birth supporting their partner. Many want to but are anxious because they have no idea what to do for the best. When I volunteered at an East London hospital on their labour ward I saw many fathers standing helplessly by, clearly wanting to be useful but really not understanding how they could best help. They looked like frightened rabbits in the headlights, always feeling like they were in the way.

The problem is, if we're around someone who is anxious and panicking we pick up on that and feel nervous and panicked ourselves. If someone is angry we start to feel angry in return. This mirroring happens automatically and unconsciously so we want to be careful about who is around us during childbirth. A woman's senses are heightened and she is likely to pick up on fear around her. If there's adrenaline and cortisol in others in the room she will start mirroring that and, much like our fellow mammals in nature, if we sense a threat around us, our body stops what it's doing until we are able to find somewhere safe to allow birth to continue undisturbed.

So the first question is, should dad be there at the birth? There are some experts, Michel Odent in particular, who feel that no, they shouldn't; he feels that a woman can't fully let go around her partner. In my experience it very much depends on the partner. The type of bond between couples and the kind of intimacy they share can vary wildly. A life partner often brings something to the birthing room that no doula, midwife, relative or friend can, and that's the understanding, trust and love that they share.

Paternal instinct is often overlooked, but can be just as powerful as the maternal instinct. It is to protect and provide. Have you ever seen gorillas giving birth in the wild? While his mate is birthing, the male gorilla will stand guard over her and nothing, but nothing, is getting past him to disturb her. That's often how I see the dads in my classes. They are tuning into an innate instinct that is 200,000 years old; it is a return to the behaviour of primitive men, men who kept guard, protecting their women from the outside world and protecting the birth of their baby. This instinct is also fuelled by hormones. Much is said about the hormonal changes in a woman's body during pregnancy and few appreciate that the same goes on for dad. About four to six weeks after a father learns there is a baby on the way his cortisol production increases. Cortisol is the stress hormone: it's his sympathetic nervous system (SNS) stepping into gear and preparing him to be on duty to protect his mate and child. About three weeks before the birth, the father's level of testosterone drops by up to a third and his prolactin level also rises, which could be nature's way of increasing his instinct to gently care for mother and baby. The male hormones return to their pre-pregnancy level about six weeks after the birth, but a father who is closely involved in the care of a baby will also experience a rise in oxytocin, that bonding instinct.

HypnoBirthing preparation for a birthing partner helps them not only to understand how a woman's body functions most effectively, but also how they can use their own instinct in the most helpful way.

> *Men: when the woman you love is being taken over by an oxytocin fuelled trip, you are going to become an adrenaline factory! Why? Because when we were hunter-gatherers she needed protecting. She still DOES! The difference now is that 'fighting' or 'fleeing' is not an option. Being present, as a protective 'force-field' of loving kindness is your job, understanding what's going on will help.* Mark Harris, midwife creator of Birthing4Blokes, in *Men, Love & Birth*

The anxiety a father feels about birth is very different from one man to another, depending on his experience and understanding. Some fathers try and disguise this anxiety by being very active during labour and birth. An anxious man is running around getting things, checking things, furiously massaging his partner, wanting to control her breathing and timing everything! Hopefully you'll have realised by now that this frantic activity is the last thing a birthing woman needs, so good preparation and information is key to being a good birthing partner. Interestingly a veterinarian in Uganda observed a gorilla giving birth in the wild; a male gorilla was seen giving the female gorilla support by sitting behind her and holding her. It's this way of channelling the supportive and protective instinct that we want to get in touch with.

While other antenatal classes will help a father or

partner understand the basics of what's going on at birth, hypnobirthing will provide a partner with a thorough understanding of the hormonal interplay and how to help create conducive conditions for the cocktail of helpful hormones needed. Often a dad will tell me that he doesn't want to see his partner in pain; he fears feeling helpless. It is important that he understands the difference between physical effort and pain. Understanding how the birthing body works builds confidence and trust in his partner's ability to birth and alleviates anxiety around such an intense experience.

Once they understand the physiological design of childbirth and the conditions optimal to its progression, partners are often the first to suggest a home birth or birthing centre. They take an active role in practising self-hypnosis techniques, they learn how to create and protect a safe space, and they take the time to equip themselves with information so they can help make informed plans and decisions. Understanding what's important to them both at the birth of their baby means he can advocate confidently, communicating their preferences to midwives and allowing his partner to focus on herself and her baby. The birthing mother is able to tune out, and retreat to the limbic part of her brain where birth exists.

Michel Odent has said, 'Many men, because they are men, are surprised and disturbed by the internal trip a woman makes to bring a child into the world,' and yes, while it can be a new experience for both parents, regular hypnosis practice means both parents are familiar with that 'no-brain' place we can take ourselves to in order to tune out distractions and focus on what is important to us. That time together strengthens their bond and sense of team and so often I meet with mothers, or receive cards, emails and calls after their baby's birth saying 'I just couldn't have done it without him'. I recently had a mum describe to me that during her baby's birth she felt like she was in a boat on the open water and sometimes the waves would be strong and powerful and she was learning to ride over them – she explained that her partner was like the lighthouse on the shoreline, a constant source of strength and comfort, keeping her focused and guiding her to safety. He reminded her to take one surge at a time when it felt overwhelming, he acknowledged her fears and yet remained confident in her ability to bring forth their baby. How wonderful.

Before the course I wasn't sure if I wanted Simon at the birth and I think if he's honest he wasn't too sure about being there! Doing the course together gave him a vital role and I wouldn't have been able to have had the experience I had without him being there. He kept me calm and relaxed me, we really worked as a team and I will never forget the feeling of having him sitting behind me supporting me as our baby was born and handed to us. Ellie

So a partner who is fully informed – knows what is going on, trusts that a woman's body is designed for birth and trusts her instinct; knows how they can best help and has practised hypnobirthing techniques with her through the pregnancy – is of huge value in the birthing room. Of course that team spirit that's created during antenatal preparation includes baby, and one of the most touching aspects of attending births, for me, has been seeing a new dad holding his baby for the first time. Tentatively figuring out how best to hold his new baby, he starts to speak and feels them relax and let go in his arms. Having spent time helping his partner focus and relax during pregnancy, his baby recognises his voice and knows she is safe. It's wonderfully moving.

Helpful hints for a hypnobirthing partner

- Oxytocin responds to feelings of love, connection, empathy and familiarity, so being tender and affectionate with your partner will really help increase oxytocin and beta-endorphins for both of you. Remember your baby was conceived through love and that same hormone will bring your baby forth too, so kissing, cuddling, privacy, massage are all incredible.
- Make the time during pregnancy to read to your partner and baby and use massage and touch to help encourage relaxation – these practices are building anchors for her to relax with your voice and touch and will prove invaluable during the birth.
- Make time during pregnancy to practise the breathing, body scans and affirmations for yourself. I've had many dads tell me how much better they're sleeping, how their work has become less stressful, and how their golf game has improved! The approach and techniques taught in hypnobirthing can be applied to all aspects of life. I even had one dad who told me it helped him pass his driving test!
- Go with your partner to the last couple of antenatal appointments. These are the ones where the subject of induction will come up and she will need you to help ask questions and convey your wishes. A 41-week pregnant woman can feel vulnerable and will benefit from your calm support.
- When labour does start, keep calm and keep smiling. There are many things about your partner's imminent behaviour that may shock and surprise you and it is important that you do not convey that to her in any way.
- If your partner feels that she can cope on her own for a

while then don't feel guilty, go to bed and get some rest. Women have been prepared for the sleep deprivation involved in labour, men have not.

- Learning how to use simple mindful tools such as breathing deeply, dropping your shoulders and lowering your voice helps keep you grounded and calm and conveys a calm, open manner to those with you during your baby's birth, rather than an adversarial form of protection.

- Encourage her to drink throughout labour and offer her food and remember to have some yourself. If your blood sugar levels drop you will be of no use to anybody, so remember to take care of yourself as well.

- When your partner's surges become intense she will need you to be strong, supportive and reassuring. With that in mind under no circumstances tell your partner (or your midwife) that 'she is tired' or that she is 'in too much pain' or 'cannot do this any longer'.

- Birth is similar mentally to running a marathon. All positive aspects must be reinforced and there is no place for negative thoughts. If you are seeing your partner in the midst of an intense surge and you are feeling overwhelmed, ask yourself this question: 'Is this upsetting my partner, can she no longer cope, or is it me that it is upsetting and can I no longer cope?' If it is the latter, remember that your partner does not have the emotional time to worry about how you are coping. Take a deep breath, relax your jaw, relax your hands and get grounded. Then, tell your partner how strong and amazing she is, because she is and she is doing all this for you and your baby.

Here are two birth stories from first-time dads who were

sceptical about hypnobirthing when told they'd been signed up for a course…

If you had told me (and Jen) 4 months ago that… 1. We'd have done a course on something called hypnobirthing, and 2. We would choose to have a home birth in a pool … I'd have called in the men in white coats.

But we did both and cannot think of a more amazing way of bringing our little man into the world. We're now passionate advocates of hypnobirthing to any friends that will listen. Anyone who knows us was puzzled when we mentioned it at first because it doesn't sound like the type of thing we would do (me being a gruff northern bloke, in particular). Not that they knew what 'it' was. Explaining hypnobirthing pre-birth, most people seemed to nod and smile and kinda see why we thought it might be useful. It's only been since Fin's arrival and the experience we had that people actually believe us… and want to know more! The proof is in the pudding and all that.

Before the course we knew as little as everyone else in our position – first-time parents who hadn't really done any in-depth reading up on what was to come. And for me, even if the birth itself had ended up being traumatic, the knowledge and confidence we got in those four sessions would have been more than worth it. Attending NCT classes a few weeks later was rather eye-opening in that most couples will have gone into labour with next to no knowledge (relatively speaking). It was difficult not to sound like a know-it-all and resist expanding on the NCT info for the other couples!

But we got much more than just the knowledge and confidence. Jen (with my help I hope… the flowering roses

89

video I put together a particular highlight) practised lots and found the positive affirmations particularly helpful. Her iPod and a 1.5hr commute each way to work definitely helped with this! And in fact I found aspects useful in work – learning to breathe properly definitely helped with anxiety and sleep!

In the comfort of our own home, in a birth pool I just about managed to pump up and fill in time, Jen was in 'established' labour for a relatively short time. We called the midwife around 9.30pm and she arrived around 10.15pm. We were so glad not to have the 'when to go to hospital?' decision and journey. Fin was born at 11.34pm. Although having cared for hypnobirthing couples before, the midwife (who was fantastic) was gobsmacked that Jen looked so good/calm/in control when she first checked her... to find she was 7cm dilated. And after 20 mins or so in the birth pool, with only a few gulps of gas and air (to focus on something rather than for pain relief it seemed), Jen was trying unsuccessfully to convince the midwife and me that the head was crowning. I even had to put my cup of tea down to check. But she was right... and a couple of contractions and some deep breaths later... POP, out he came (it was that easy, surely?! :)). Jen said later she didn't feel as though she particularly had to do anything – her body and Fin were in control and knew what to do.

Awestruck/lost for words/dumbfounded... I can't quite find the right phrase for what I felt. We kept him attached to the cord and in the water with Jen for 20 mins or so, before I grabbed him for some chest-hair-eating time. Jen was taken for a shower and a check and was tucked up in our own bed within the hour. Perfect. Rick

This was our first child and being a man I didn't know what to expect with regards the pregnancy period and the birth.

The role of the man up to and during the birth has always been portrayed as a hapless onlooker who wants nothing to do with the messy and faint-inducing business of giving birth. My own father was playing cricket when he heard my mother had gone into labour and decided that the cricket team needed him more than my mother did.

Attitudes among my generation do seem to be changing though and when my wife said she had enrolled us onto a hypnobirthing course I was open-minded but didn't know what to expect (actually I half-expected a bunch of 'yogurt weavers', as my brother calls them). However, I was very glad she did as from the very first class I felt much more at ease and more involved knowing that I had a role to play and wasn't a mere onlooker.

When Kat (my wife) started labour we were both calm and relieved that it was finally happening. We had decided early on that we wanted a home birth and I had found an inflatable birthing pool on the internet to set up in our living room. We had friends take the dog and went for a walk round the block. This was early evening and by about 9.30pm the contractions were such that it was time to call the midwife. Two of them promptly came at about 11pm and I set about making cups of tea and filling up the birth pool to the desired temperature. The two midwives were lovely with a kind manner and didn't get in the way or try and dictate things at all. The CD of hypno music was playing and I rubbed Kat's back for what seemed like three hours while she did her breathing. Kat wanted to try and avoid the *use of any drugs or gas and to experience the birth as naturally as possible. After more cups of tea and rounds of sandwiches Kat was ready to get into the pool at about 4am. I sat on the side holding her hand and whispering encouragement.*

First came the head then the rest just whooshed out into the water shortly after. Instead of the baby being whipped away and checked we wanted to hold her straight away and I watched in amazement as Kat held this tiny wrinkled baby in her arms and cried with relief and joy. I was not really prepared for the afterbirth and I would suggest to any men reading this that they can probably skip this bit. It was painful for Kat and at this point she did reach for the gas. Kat ended up with a few stitches which the midwives dealt with but it was nothing serious. After the midwives made their checks we bade them farewell and they left us alone with this new life that we had created. The sun was coming up and we were high on lack of sleep and elation. We announced the birth to friends and family then lay side-by-side in bed with a glass of champagne and a silly grin on our faces knowing our family had begun and life would never be the same again. Richard

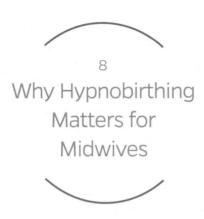

8

Why Hypnobirthing Matters for Midwives

A midwife or obstetrician needs to understand how the energy of childbirth flows; to not know is to be like a physicist who doesn't understand about gravity.

Ina May Gaskin

I've thought long and hard about this chapter. I'm aware of the fine line between wanting to share information and running the risk of sounding patronising, which is far from my intention. Thankfully, there are some midwives working within the NHS who've trained in hypnobirthing and with more and more NHS hospitals offering HypnoBirthing classes awareness continues to grow. Midwives are seeing hypnobirthing parents more and more often. However, having only recently had a client tell me that when she told her midwife she was doing HypnoBirthing she replied 'Oh, that's that thing with the little pills, isn't it?' I think there's perhaps still some work to be done.

I should say right away that I have enormous respect for midwives and, on the whole, we're extremely lucky to have the system of midwifery that we do in the UK. The word midwife comes from an Old English term meaning 'with woman', which reflects the traditional midwife's role of waiting for nature and supporting a woman during pregnancy and birth. The French term for midwife, *sage-femme* ('wise woman') is equally insightful. To be 'with woman' is to get to know her through pregnancy, help support her and alleviate her concerns and fears. Being 'with woman' during labour and birth is to best understand how she is progressing through her behaviour and demeanour rather than clinical exams and stopwatches. Sadly most pregnant women do not have an assigned midwife to support them throughout pregnancy, but meet many antenatally and more still during labour.

Dr Dick-Read's fascination with the riddle of why some women feel pain during labour and others didn't guided his entire career. As a medical student watching experienced midwives he noticed that sometimes women who came to the London Hospital in the agony of a difficult labour could be eased and soothed by the attention of a sympathetic midwife. A midwife could go to a woman who had been the 'picture of agony and torture', stroke her hair and talk to her in such a way that the pain, if not the effort, would seem to disappear. It's well documented how continuous, caring, non-judgemental support helps a labouring woman feel safe and be able to let go – thereby producing the most helpful hormones and easing birth. The medical model of birth has become so entrenched in many busy labour wards, however, that the simplest and most effective ways of helping women give birth are in danger of being lost.

> *I don't think we are adding anything very useful to the birthing process myself. The mother has all that is needed for that, she is to be worshipped in that sense. Anything we offer should be just that, an offering, which she takes*

or leaves dependent on her whim! We may be adding some stuff, but it's worth little if we don't have faith in her magnificence. Mark Harris, midwife

It's important that our midwives, our guardians of 'normal' birth, see undisturbed births and are reacquainted with the intelligence of the human body in giving birth. We need more of what Michel Odent calls 'authentic midwives' – experienced birth attendants who can recognise the stage of labour without repeating vaginal exams, just by listening to the noise a labouring woman is making, watching her posture and observing the expression on her face. This patient, instinctive approach to being 'with woman' is, worryingly, in danger of being lost among the machines, routine procedures and administration of hospitals and even birthing centres. The most common complaint I hear from experienced midwives who've been practising for decades is that it used to be that birth was seen to be normal until it wasn't; whereas now the approach seems to be that it is abnormal until it can be proven to be normal. With the increase in tests, charts and boxes to be ticked it's easy to slip unwittingly into a mindset in which if a woman or baby doesn't fit a preordained idea of what is 'normal', then something must be done. Our idea of 'normal', however, changes. In the 1970s the medicalisation of childbirth was possibly at its peak, with the power of midwifery at its lowest ebb. It was the norm for birth to take place in a sterile hospital room, and for nurses and doctors to wear masks. Episiotomies were routine, and it was normal for the baby to be hung upside-down after birth, be slapped to make it breathe and then almost immediately afterwards taken from its mother to be washed, dressed and bottle-fed in a nursery. Thankfully times have changed but there's still a way to go.

Possibly the most famous midwife in the world, Ina May

Gaskin, talks of the vow of a midwife to put the welfare of the mother and the child first – that is, above herself and above the policies of the institution in which she works. In an increasingly risk-averse and medico-legal culture, midwives are coming under great pressure to conform to rigidly prescriptive obstetric protocols. Yet many women still want the type of care that falls outside standard guidelines – they may want to have a vaginal birth after caesarean (VBAC) at home, to give birth to a baby presenting by the breech or to avoid caesarean delivery of twins. Hypnobirthing couples are given the information and confidence to stand up for themselves and their babies when they feel standardised 'box ticking' care just isn't good enough, and we need midwives to stand by their side. Working together you make a formidable team!

> *The more births I attend, the more I realise how much I disturb the birthing woman. Disturbing often comes disguised in the form of 'helping'. Asking the mother questions, constant verbal coaching, side conversations in the room, clicking cameras – there are so many ways to draw the mother from her ancient brain trance (necessary for a smooth expulsion of the baby) into the present-time world (using the neo-cortex which interferes with smooth birth). This must be avoided.* Gloria Lemay, birth attendant

So for midwives, doulas and all birth workers working with couples who've prepared for birth using hypnosis, here are some helpful hints for working together:

- Help keep the birthing environment calm and peaceful: enter the room quietly, keep lights dim, speak softly, keep noise and chatter and the presence of staff to a minimum. A mother will want to retreat to her birthing space within and has practised doing so with self-hypnosis. You can help this by avoiding asking her questions and interrupting her focus. Speak with her partner in the first instance.

- Your own attitude cannot be ignored: how you are feeling, talking and behaving will have an effect on birth. Use gentle, positive language: words like 'intense' and 'powerful' are appropriate; there is however a distinction to be made between pain and physical effort, so do not use the word 'pain', or suggest something may 'sting', 'hurt', or 'be uncomfortable' or 'difficult'. Words are powerfully suggestive, so focus on using only positive language. You can use gentler words such as 'surge' instead of 'contraction', or 'breathe baby down' instead of 'push'.
- Encourage the use of breathing: hypnobirthing breathing involves long, deep, slow breaths which help mum and baby remain calm, and mum to remain in control of each surge.
- Cover the clock and any other technical equipment not required.
- Read and respect the parents' birth preferences. Discuss any issues in a gentle and encouraging way. You can be sure a hypnobirthing couple have researched and discussed their wishes together, and have made their decisions after considered thought.
- If a recommended intervention needs to be discussed, speak to dad/birth partner first, quietly away from mum, in order to keep mum's stress levels at a minimum. They can then calmly discuss options as a couple. You may find that they ask for more information, particularly around the benefits and risks of suggested procedures. Calm, reasoned information and advice is much appreciated.

- Please do not tell a mum she will need a specific pain relief (epidural, etc). Wait for her to ask if she needs it. You can rest assured that hypnobirthing parents are well aware of what is available and will ask for help if they feel they need it. Drugs are not a dirty word with hypnobirthing preparation, but their use is an informed one and it is not for anybody else to assume they know what a birthing woman is experiencing. Women are highly suggestible while in labour and to suggest they might need something can plant a suggestion where it is not needed.

- Avoid coaching mum to 'push', unless it is absolutely necessary. Encourage mum to follow her body's urges to bear down as they come and encourage her to 'breathe the baby down the birth path'. If the jaw is clenched then the pelvis is tense, and if the jaw is opened and soft then the pelvis relaxes and opens out. Ina May Gaskin calls this the 'sphincter law' and she has found that a relaxed mouth and jaw directly correlate with the ability of the cervix and vagina to soften and open fully. Following this principle it is possible to breathe the baby out rather than actively push. This knowledge has not been a part of routine medical practice, where the Valsalva manoeuvre of closing the mouth, pursing the lips and straining down on the pelvis is often advised by traditionalists. Breathing a baby down and out is a key component to pregnancy hypnosis courses and is often not taught in standard antenatal classes.

- You can trust a woman who says her baby is coming, even if she appears calm and quiet! Even the most experienced of midwives can be surprised by how calm and confident a hypnobirthing couple can be, especially when expecting their first baby.

We LOVE hypnobirthing! More and more of our clients are using it and we always discuss it as a resource when we book our clients and explain the huge benefits to both parents and babies. Of course as midwives who have more ways of assessing a labour than just vaginal examinations, it can be a bit tricky to accurately gauge where a woman is in her labour when she is hypnobirthing. There has been more than one occasion when I arrived at a labour and thought 'This woman isn't in labour!' only to be surprised by a baby's arrival an hour later! Jacqui Tomkins, *British Journal of Midwifery* Midwife of the Year, 2014

Many thanks to Vanessa Hodge, a midwife on a high-risk labour ward and hypnobirthing teacher, for the following suggestions:

- Midwives need to learn to do their newborn examination while the baby is skin-to-skin! The entire examination can be done with baby on mum's chest or abdomen, the administration of Vitamin K, temperature, measuring: baby can be lifted onto the scales next to mum for the few seconds it take to weigh them. This way bonding is preserved and baby is kept warm too!
- Hypnobirthing is not just for normal, natural births – it is for every type of birth and should not be disregarded or dismissed by staff when a natural birth becomes more complex. An example of this would be when transfer from a low-risk area (home or birth centre) to a high-risk labour ward is required. It is at this point that hypnobirthing will make a huge difference to the woman's feeling of control, and her ability to stay calm in an emergency or medicalised birth.
- Think about how you can keep the room calm and quiet even in an emergency. If it is a ventouse or forceps

the room's main lights can be off or dimmed and music can still play. The spotlight can be on the area the doctor is looking at and working in and we do not need every light in the room on. Noise can be kept to a minimum and any unnecessary staff can be outside the room.

- Let us as midwives keep families together. Why can the partner and baby not go to theatre with mum for a routine third degree tear repair, or manual removal of the placenta? The dad and baby would be in theatre for an instrumental birth or a c-section under regional analgesia. Why are we separating mother, father and baby after the birth, in order to carry out a routine procedure in theatre? I always offer for the father and the baby to go too. Mum can then have skin-to-skin in theatre and dad can be there to hold baby if she feels unwell at any time. It is vitally important to keep families together after the birth. This way the procedure is not significant for the woman as she is distracted by gazing at, cuddling and bonding with her baby and almost forgets why she is in theatre. Afterwards she just remembers a lovely time in theatre cuddling her baby and not the procedure itself and the sadness and loss of not being with her baby.

A midwife's birth story

I knew very little about hypnobirthing until I started the course. From the little knowledge and very minimal experience I had of it (one very quick home birth) I thought it was about using relaxation techniques, although I didn't know what these were, to hopefully achieve a natural birth with no pain-relieving drugs.

I now realise there is so much more to it, the use of your partner's touch, finding your own ways to relax e.g. familiar smells and music, thinking positively and ensuring a calm environment. I didn't realise before that there is actually quite a lot of preparation involved. I also didn't realise how much time I would invest in learning to calm myself and relax.

Having done hypnobirthing will definitely change some of the ways I practise. When talking through labour with women I will spend more time discussing breathing and relaxation techniques. At births I will try to ensure as calm and quiet an environment as possible. I remember being so grateful for a darkened room. We had one small light on for the midwife to see what she was doing and I remember that every time I moved around in the pool, the midwife moved the light away from me, which was so thoughtful of her. One of the most important things explained to us during the course was stating in our birth plan for no pain relief to be offered. I can really see why this is so important. Had I been offered any I would have thought that I wasn't coping and should probably have something, then the experience would have been completely different. I will never suggest pain relief again! Women know it's there if they need it.

Unfortunately, a lot of my colleagues don't have much time for hypnobirthing. I assume they think it's all about hypnotising someone. Even those midwives who do have time for it really don't understand it. One asked me the other day if I 'did the hypnobirthing' during the birth, so I tried to explain that it's not really about doing one specific thing at that time, but utilising all or some of the techniques you've learned leading up to the birth. So I suppose if you can get across that it's not like the hypnotising you might see on a TV programme then my colleagues might have a bit more time for it!

When I return to work I will definitely talk about hypnobirthing and try to encourage my colleagues to look into it more. My friends and family have become very interested in it having heard I had a drug-free birth. I didn't tell everyone that I was doing the course as I didn't want sceptics to make negative comments, so it's very satisfying to now be able to say that yes, it really does work. Ellie, hypnobirthing mother and practising midwife

> *You are a midwife.*
> *You are assisting at someone else's birth*
> *Do good without show or fuss.*
> *Facilitate what is happening*
> *rather than what you think*
> *ought to be happening.*
> *If you must, take the lead.*
> *Lead so that the mother is helped,*
> *yet still free and in charge.*
> *When the babe is born*
> *the mother will rightly say,*
> *'We did it ourselves'*

Lao Tzu, *Tao Te Ching*, 5th century BC

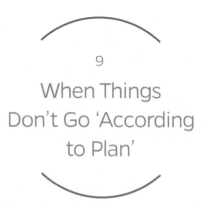

9

When Things Don't Go 'According to Plan'

Remaining in control in labour and birth means being able to adapt calmly and peacefully to a sometimes rapidly changing situation, having the ability to refocus at each twist and turn without fear or distress but with calmness and confidence.

Vanessa Hodge, midwife and hypnobirthing teacher

By learning hypnobirthing methods, mothers-to-be can discover how to manage tensions that are caused by fear, helping to avoid pain and discomfort. Hypnobirthing prepares both mind and body to work the way nature intended, and even where special medical circumstances might arise, hypnobirthing helps birthing mothers to feel calmer and more in control when faced with decisions about treatment options. It truly is about being prepared for any and all birth experiences.

I have become increasingly concerned that there may be a misunderstanding that a hypnobirth has to look and sound a certain way (at home, in the dark, in water and completely silent). Certainly a lot of hypnobirthing mums do opt for home birth, as they instinctively feel safest there, which is the most important thing for a woman in labour. When she and her partner are armed with information and prepared, they know that a home birth will give her a greater chance of avoiding intervention. For some women, however, a birthing centre offers midwife-led care within a hospital and that gives them comfort. Some women don't have the option, either because of lack of resources in the area or because of medical conditions that require her to be supported more closely. Circumstances can change during birth too, of course. Some of the most empowered, beautiful births I've attended have been in labour ward rooms and the operating theatre. The beauty of self-hypnosis is that it's portable. It travels with you and so the techniques you've practised throughout pregnancy will help you wherever and however your baby is born.

A positive birth means a birth in which a woman feels she has freedom of choice, access to accurate information, and that she is in control, powerful and respected. A birth that she approaches, perhaps with some trepidation, but without fear or dread, and that she then goes on to enjoy, and later remember with warmth and pride.

A positive birth does not have to be 'natural' or 'drug-free' – it simply has to be informed from a place of positivity as opposed to fear. You can birth with positivity in hospital or at home, with or without medical intervention. You can have a positive caesarean, or a positive home water birth. Positive Birth is about approaching birth realistically, having genuine choice, and feeling empowered by your experience. Milli Hill, founder of the Positive Birth Movement

Women who feel let down by their birth experience often worry that they have failed. They may feel they have missed out on that sense of empowerment and strength that some women discuss when telling birth stories, and this can lead to feelings of insecurity. The truth is, however, that birth can sometimes be unpredictable. There are two of you involved in this journey and your baby hasn't read the books you've read or attended the classes you have (well they have, but in a different way!) and may have ideas of her own. There are so many variables that can affect childbirth, so perhaps we do best to control those we can and understand those we can't. All women have inner strength, and accepting a change in a birth plan requires courage and understanding.

In my psychotherapy training I specialised in Rational Emotive Behaviour Therapy (REBT), a trans-diagnostic, evidence-based strand of cognitive behavioural therapy developed by Albert Ellis in the 1950s. Based on ancient Stoic philosophy it teaches us that it's not what happens to us that causes disturbance, but the thoughts we have about what happens, or doesn't.

Specifically, Albert Ellis maintained that as human beings we take what we'd like to have happen – for instance: 'I'd like my baby to be born naturally, at home' and automatically, and unknowingly, elevate it into a demand: 'I *must* birth my baby naturally, at home', the knock-on effect of which is a feeling that 'If I don't have my baby naturally at home then I've failed as a woman, everyone will judge me, they'll think badly of me and I'll feel like a failure'.

Think about it; we do this to ourselves most of the time. We turn preferences into demands that are so loaded we will punish ourselves if we fail to achieve them: 'I must do this presentation perfectly; if I don't they'll think I'm rubbish and I can't bear that, it would be the end of the world and everyone will think I'm a failure,' rather than 'I'd really like this presentation to go well, I accept it may not be perfect but I'll do my best, this alone has no bearing on whether I'm a success or failure.' We need to focus on what we'd *like* to have happen, while acknowledging the possibility that it might not.

This is why, rather than writing a birth *plan*, with hypnobirthing we discuss birth *preferences*. In an ideal world, how would you like things to be when you welcome your baby into the world? Where do you want to be, who do you want around you and how would you prefer they treat you? In addition to the techniques taught with hypnobirthing preparation the information shared about birthing options and hospital procedures is done with care and consideration. All too often NHS and NCT classes are information channels for local hospitals, so they teach a birth preparation class that is primarily designed to acquaint you with the medical model. They educate you about the drugs, technological apparatus and hospital procedure. In short they are teaching you how to be a good, acquiescing patient. With hypnobirthing understanding the conditions that will allow you to feel safe and comfortable, encourage helpful hormones and inhibit unhelpful hormones means you can start to prepare a 'wish list' specifically for you. You will discuss all aspects of birth: induction of labour, the birth environment, 'routine' procedures during labour, birth positions, cord clamping, skin-to-skin contact, delivery of the placenta, Vitamin K and more – you will be able to discuss all these things with your partner so you can figure out together what's important to you. This is crucial too for your partner to feel confident as your advocate during birth. The last thing a birthing mother needs is to be answering questions and 'thinking' about anything; she can focus inwards when she knows her wishes have been, and will be, clearly expressed and followed.

As Milli Hill says:

> Women can often be discouraged from preparing for birth or making any kind of plan. 'Just go with the flow', they are told, 'Birth is unpredictable, you can't control it'. This is true, to an extent. But the danger with this attitude is that it encourages women to be completely passive in their birth experience and place themselves and what happens to them completely in the hands of others. Unfortunately, in the current birth climate, this can mean that choices are made for them in the heat of labour that they would not have made themselves, and it is only with the luxury of retrospect that they can then think, 'If only I had had a say'.
>
> While you cannot control birth itself, you can control aspects of it. You can control your own emotions and fears with sound preparation. You can know your human rights. You can set the bar of how you expect to be treated. You can control the atmosphere in the birth room. You can make clear your wishes for how you want to labour, deliver, and what you need to happen in the moments after birth.
>
> Hypnobirthing matters because it sets women on a journey to take charge of their births. It gives the message that birth preparation is vital and essential for a positive birth, both for spiralling inwards and finding strength and courage, and for making and voicing decisions that feel right about the outer environment in labour and birth.

Hypnobirthing is about complete antenatal preparation. Every intervention in the normal process of birth introduces risks as well as benefits. When interventions become routine rather than judiciously used the balance tips towards risks rather than benefits, because one intervention tends to lead to another and often produces a cascade effect. For example, continuous monitoring (CTG) confines women to bed, which can slow labour down. Doctors may then want to give artificial oxytocin (syntocinon), which increases pain, causing women to want an epidural. The epidural can slow labour or cause abnormal heart rate patterns, ending the cascade in caesarean section for poor progress or fetal distress.

One of the most common fears couples come to me with is that they will be swept along by medical intervention, not understand what is going on and feel they have no choice. Nothing could be further from the truth. This is your baby, your body and your birth. In the UK nobody is able to do anything unless you give permission. Sadly options aren't often explicitly made clear and many people are surprised when we start discussing options and weighing up risks and benefits so each couple can feel equipped to make informed decisions. With hypnobirthing it is not about learning to become a good patient, but becoming a good parent. Good parents want to find the optimal conditions for bringing their baby safely and joyously into the world, and they are not willing to settle for anything less.

'I wish I had known that when I was pregnant'

Obstetric interventions that can be used for convenience rather than necessity, such as induction of labour, epidurals and continuous fetal monitoring, unintentionally put women on a conveyor belt to medicalised birth, leading them away from the possibility of natural birth and all the benefits that brings. Research has shown that feeling in control during childbirth is associated with positive feelings about birth experiences, while women who do not feel in control of their birth have higher levels of dissatisfaction and may experience long-term psychological trauma.

It has been said to me, 'But you have to trust them, they're doctors'. It's not about doubting or belittling the high levels of training and skill our midwives and doctors have, but hypnobirthing dares to suggest you put your trust in yourself. In your body, in your baby and in your instinct. When left to start and progress undisturbed birth will, more often than not, proceed without incident. If procedures are offered – and the language of childbirth often feels more like instruction than an offer – then the ability to remain calm, ask questions and weigh up the benefits and risks of all options means parents-to-be are able to make informed decisions that feel right for them and their baby. It is about avoiding unnecessary intervention and being grateful for help when it's needed. This in turn has been shown to result in a positive attitude to birth, however it progresses.

To demonstrate that hypnobirthing is for all eventualities, there follow various birth stories where things didn't necessarily go 'to plan', and hypnobirthing preparation proved invaluable. The hypnobirthing books and courses will provide information about each of these scenarios and help you ask questions to weigh up risks and benefits. If you need help during your pregnancy and birth there are organisations who can support you with information and advice, such as AIMS, IMUK and Birthrights. Contact details are at the back of the book. Working with a trained hypnobirthing professional will ensure you get individual care and they can also signpost local help for you.

Induction of labour

One thing is certain – choosing to induce labour will totally alter your birth experience and the options open to you. It can be difficult to untangle and isolate the risks involved with induction because usually more than one risk factor is occurring at once: for instance, if chemicals are used to stimulate labour, then continuous monitoring is also required, which restricts movement. Often an epidural is also in place. All of these carry their own risks.

Couples are always surprised to hear that they can decline induction of labour. The language of permission entrenched in pregnancy and childbirth is such that you'll often hear, from your very first appointment, 'We'll let you go to 40+10 days (this time frame changes depending on your hospital trust's policy) and then we'll induce you.' Notice the 'We'll let you'… any permission is given from you rather than the hospital and once equipped with information and genuine confidence that the baby will come when they are ready many parents are happy to wait patiently. Those that agree to induction do so with good reason and are calm, confident and approach it optimistically. This seems to make the world of difference.

My due date came and went, and at 40+5 we went in for a routine check-up. Immediately my midwife tried to book me in for an induction. When we asked about alternatives she told me my placenta would start to die at 40 weeks. My 'hypno hackles' went up – that's simply not true; your placenta can start to deteriorate at any time and 'die' is an emotive word to use on a pregnant lady. I said we would be happy to be booked in for induction at the latest date the hospital offered (40+13) as long as I could see a consultant before then. I was given an appointment for a consultant at 40+12. I was offered a sweep by the midwife, who seemed resigned when I turned it down! I walked out of the room feeling massively empowered and even the midwife was impressed by my stats from hypnobirthing and personal research.

The weekend came and went with no baby. I took walks, had acupuncture, ate well and rested. I also cried and swore at everyone phoning about my progress – it's a hugely emotional time and everyone has an opinion, and they aren't afraid to share it.

We went to see the consultant, ready for battle. We needn't have worried. While the midwife we saw first was horrified at our stance, the consultant was sympathetic and listened to our point of view. We saw her on a Tuesday and after a liquor scan to check the baby had enough fluid she said we were fine to proceed with monitoring. I had a sweep, as I was curious to see if my body had started any sort of labour preparation. Hearing I was 1cm was a huge boost, as was the consultant predicting I'd go into labour naturally. I cancelled my induction, booked in some additional monitoring, and also another induction for the following Monday – I wanted to know all options were available to me.

At lunchtime on 40+13 I had my first mild contraction, six hours after the time my induction appointment had been. That evening I had a couple of glasses of wine and went to bed. At 2am I couldn't sleep through my contractions so took a bath, and at 3.30am I woke my husband and we watched comedy, stuck on the tens machine and did some massage. A black cab (ideal for labour – the yellow disability bars are fab) took us through the streets of Hackney at dawn to the hospital. On arrival at the hospital we were told to wait in the waiting room as they were full. Embarrassed about the mooing noises and movement I was using with each strong contraction I waited in the corridor, alone, while my husband badgered the reception midwife for an examination. This was the lowest point. I was in pain, alone, and frightened of being

*sent home. I found a bathroom and was discovered –
mooing and moving – by a midwife. 'We'd better take a
look at you,' she said. My waters broke on examination
and she confirmed I was 10cm – no wonder my labour
was more full-on than the quieter ladies in the waiting
room! She told me she'd be off shift in an hour and would
come and meet my baby. She was slightly optimistic –
Arthur was born an hour and 45 mins later, with help
from wonderful midwives – their advice on position
really helped, as did their encouragement. He weighed
7lb 8oz (3.4kg) and came out with lots of hair on his
head, but no signs at all of being overcooked. He is a
happy baby, with no extended crying – and he's gorgeous!*

*This was right for me. Make the decision that works
for you – that may include induction!! While I laboured
with no drugs (which had been my plan), if I hadn't
arrived so late I would have taken them – I don't believe
it would have been at odds with my hypno experience,
it would have been another decision I could have made
for me and my labour, enabled by hypno. It's not about
whale music and a zen labour – it's about what's right
for you and ensuring you have the tools and information
to own the experience, however that may go.* Anna

*I didn't quite get the Hypnobirth I had hoped for as I had
to be induced at 41 weeks and 1 day. My baby had very
little fluid left around her, her heart rate was a concern
and my placenta had started to calcify. Once you know
there are medical concerns the most important thing is
getting the baby out safely. We could have gone straight
to a room after the check-up, but as it was so unexpected
I felt confident enough to ask for an hour to return home
and collect my things and mentally prepare.*

I had been really nervous about having an induction but the staff at the hospital were amazing and I had a midwife who had practised hypnobirthing so I was able to use it as much as I could. The main frustration was not being able to move around as I was wired up to the drip and the monitor. However, my husband got the room atmosphere relaxed and as it was evening it felt very calm. I think I used my MP3s through the majority of the labouring and although I could never get into my blissful state I knew the tracks so well it was really comforting to have something so familiar playing in my ear and helping me through. The breathing techniques were invaluable and to be honest I don't know how I would have managed without the hypnobirthing.

In the end I was about 10 hours from the drip going in to our baby being born. I only used a tens machine until just before I was ready to push and then gas and air. I think they were amazed I didn't have an epidural, as I think it is more common when you have been induced. The wave breath was great, together with the golden thread and ocean's breath from yoga it got me though every surge.

She was very relaxed when she came out, crawled to the breast and fed straightaway and is quite a chilled out baby.
Lynn

Breech baby

The vast majority of babies instinctively turn head down in preparation for birth. If a baby hasn't done this by 36 weeks, various options will be offered to help encourage a baby to turn. The most effective natural methods to help turn a baby are hypnosis and acupuncture.

A study in 1992 by Dr Lewis Mehl-Madrona ended with 81 of the 100 breech babies having turned spontaneously from breech to vertex (head down) presentation with hypnosis and visualisation. In the comparison group of 100 women who did not participate in hypnotherapy, only 26 babies turned spontaneously. It was originally thought that each mother would require approximately ten hours of hypnotherapy in order to accomplish the desired result. As the study unfolded, the average number of hours with each woman was only four, and half of the successful 81 turns required only one session.

For some babies it's simply not right for them to turn: they know what's right for them and it's not uncommon for babies who have been forcibly turned by ECV (external cephalic version, a procedure where baby is physically manipulated into the head-down position) to flip right back around again. Sadly the NHS no longer routinely trains midwives in catching breech babies born vaginally, so a caesarean section is often given as the only option for birth. Hypnobirthing, naturally, encourages you to look at all options.

At 38 weeks pregnant I hired independent midwives to help me have a physiological breech birth at home because the NHS were not supportive of my choices and wanted me to opt for a caesarean. I came across the wonderful Maya midwives, who happened to be experienced in vaginal breech birth and very keen to support me. I was overjoyed and it meant there was a greater chance I could have the home birth I so desperately wanted. I withdrew from NHS care and had regular visits from the midwives, and then it was just a waiting game. I began listening to my Natal Hypnotherapy CD again every day, sometimes two or three times a day, and I made a poster for my bedroom wall with affirmations and other positive thoughts about the birth.

My due date came and went and a week later there were still no labour signs. The midwives advised that I didn't do anything to augment the labour, such as acupuncture or reflexology, because breech babies must come when they are ready. So I waited. Natal Hypnotherapy helped me to remain calm, relaxed and focused, when friends and family were growing increasingly concerned. When I reached 42 weeks I decided to go to hospital for a scan and CTG monitoring to make sure everything was ok. The doctors said baby was doing really well and couldn't find anything wrong, but that they would be happier if I'd have a c-section the next day.

My instincts told me to wait so I agreed to come back two days later for more monitoring. In the meantime I began to prepare myself for a caesarean by listening to the Natal Hypnotherapy CD. Again the CTG monitoring showed that everything was fine, but I agreed to go in the next day for my bloods to be taken in case the caesarean was necessary. Although I was more prepared for it, I couldn't understand how my body could grow this baby, keep her nourished for nine months and then just abandon her and me when it was time to be born.

That night I woke at 4am with contractions that felt 'different' to the Braxton Hicks I'd been having for weeks so I called the midwife, Andy. I wasn't in any pain but had been preparing for this for months using Natal Hypnotherapy so didn't really expect to be. During the labour itself I listened to a CD of relaxing birth music which triggered my relaxation. I then focused on deep breathing down to my baby and visualising during contractions. There was about an hour where the contractions were really intense but at no time painful and our daughter was born two and a half hours later, bum first, at 7.30am. As the birth was so quick there was no time to get in the pool or do anything else I had planned! Andy said it was the quickest birth she'd ever seen, so quick that Viv, the second *midwife, missed it! I was glad I called Andy when I did. Our beautiful breech baby daughter, Amália Rose, was born calmly and peacefully in our bedroom, 17 days past the due date. I couldn't have hoped for a better outcome, I am so glad that I trusted my instincts and my baby and that I had the support of such wonderful midwives.* Ruth

Caesarean birth

Sometimes a caesarean birth is truly necessary and we can be grateful that this life-saving technology has become so much safer and more accessible for women around the world. Having a good caesarean requires forethought and, especially in the event of a planned, more family-centred c-section, a good relationship with caregivers who are open to discussion and negotiation. Hypnobirthing helps you with this planning, gives you the tools to remain calm in the lead up to and throughout birth and helps ensure a swift recovery afterwards.

My birth was a more planned affair than expected. Scans highlighted a placenta praevia which we monitored up to the last weeks, but it didn't move and a date was set in the diary for our baby's arrival.

My 'due date' fell on Easter Sunday and we were booked in for a week before that. It was advised that it would be dangerous for me to go into labour and for the placenta to come before the baby. However, with NHS rules dictating that with a placenta praevia there should be one consultant present in theatre, the date was brought forward another week on account of them all being away for the Easter break! Initially I was a little thrown by this, but with a few moments of Hypnobirthing breathing and a bit of regrounding I decided that this was fine... baby was ready and a good weight, I was ready (and huge) and

I felt fortunate to still have a little time to wrap up my last bits of work. At least I had some time left to prepare.

I contacted our teacher who helped us to adapt our birth partner script and hypnobirthing tools and I got into a good routine of daily meditation and relaxation, even having a little chat with baby, explaining what was happening and when we would meet each other. I also began to visualise all the people that would be involved in my care and in her safe delivery, surrounding the situation with loving, positive thoughts. By the time the day came I was filled with happy anticipation and excitement.

Our anaesthetist was an amazing man, totally calm and reassuring. I had the Hippo Instrumental playing on my phone close to my head. I became a bit shivery and nervous as the cannula appeared, but amazed them with my recovery with a few more hypno moves and using the lavender stick. We were calmly talked through the operation: when it began, when baby was close to arriving and when things were concluding. I had asked not to be given any more detail than that.

It was the most peaceful, magical, amazing experience I could have had and I will never forget it. Eloise was eased out (no tools!) and lifted up to see us, alert but calm. She gave a cry and coughed up the fluid from the lungs. These were two things we had been told she might need help with; she didn't! Her Apgar score was 9 out of 10 in the first minute. They promptly wrapped her (operating theatres can be chilly) and it felt as though she was with me almost instantaneously, calm and on my chest, looking up at us both, before she went in to a calm sleep. Cord clamping was delayed and I had plenty of time with her before she went with daddy to be weighed and checked again. I felt huge elation, as well as a mist of calm and serene acceptance that my long journey had finally concluded with the joyful outcome we had striven for. Sarah

Twins born naturally

Women who are expecting twins or higher-order multiples often wonder if they will be able to have a vaginal birth or if they will be required to have a caesarean section. Well, as long as your labour is uncomplicated, it is entirely possible (and usually recommended) to birth both babies vaginally. As with all births it requires preparation and a supportive team around you.

If you're expecting more than one baby join TAMBA (Twins and Multiple Birth Association tamba.org.uk) for information and support to help you prepare for life with your babies.

Here's a beautiful birth story from Tracey, who birthed her twin daughters having used hypnosis in preparation.

I always dreamt of having twins but never thought that it would become a reality. After a difficult year of fertility treatment I got pregnant. At 40 weeks and two days my labour started spontaneously. I felt a pop and excitedly woke my husband. It was strange as I was sure my membranes had released, but there was no water in sight. Once at the hospital I was pleased to see the birthing room I wanted was free. It was spacious with a large birthing pool and natural landscape on the wall. At this point we called Tamara, our doula and friend.

The next few hours passed peacefully. I had dimmed lights, relaxing music and the two most important people with me – my husband Ben and my doula. They were a great support system and stopped any unnecessary interruptions. The pressure in my back was getting stronger and stronger so my doula advised that I keep changing positions. I started in a standing position, swaying side to side with my husband as my pillar of support. Before long I felt sleepy and so decided to lean over my birthing ball and here I rocked peacefully while my husband massaged my back. My doula added a heat pack and it was such a relief. I even snoozed for a little while!

At around 6am I asked to get into the birthing pool, but after checking my dilation the midwife on duty didn't feel that I was far enough into established labour. This happened with my first pregnancy too. If you are calm people often assume you are not very far on, but I just knew things would increase rapidly from that moment on. My doula was very supportive and said, 'just remember it is just a number, you are doing great'. By the time the midwives changed morning shifts I was in the pool. I felt urges to bear down and the pressure in my back was becoming more intense and very different to what I had experienced with my first birth – I now know that this was probably because Emily was back to back. I continued to use my hypnobirthing breaths in between surges to stay calm and relaxed. My new midwife was amazing. She had experience of natural twin birth and immediately put me at ease with her confidence and calm persona. She could see that my labour was progressing quickly and requested I get out of the pool for some intermittent monitoring, but gave me the option to return if I wanted to. I was offered gas and air and used it to change positions.

By about 8.30am I was upright on the bed, leaning over my ball. I made some humming noises and practised my surge breaths as I rocked back and forth and this helped me to continue to stay calm and relaxed. Another hour passed and I decided to lean over the back of the bed. Being in this upright position felt comfortable and I was able to rest *a little between surges. They were coming very frequently now and I was advised that I was fully dilated.*

At 10.21am Emily Grace was birthed gently into the world weighing 7lb 5oz (3.3kg). She didn't make a sound, but instead just looked up at me. She was so calm and relaxed, yet so alert. I was able to hold her while I waited for her cord to stop pulsating. Staring into her little face was the most amazing feeling.

Five minutes passed and my surges had yet to return. I was asked to turn around and was shocked to find a room full of medical professionals. I was so deep in self-hypnosis that I had no idea that they were there! After a further ten minutes I could see that the medical professionals were getting uneasy and they had started to prepare a drip. After getting through my entire labour without any interference I was reluctant to let it happen now. My doula advised that I try latching Emily on to the breast as this might help. I started to feel some mild surges and my husband and Tamara helped me get back into the upright position. Ben held my hand and told me that I was doing great and that he was so proud of me. Tamara held Emily so I knew she was in safe hands.

Within less than five minutes Eryn Rose's head was birthed. This time it felt so fast. Eryn was in the perfect birthing position with her waters intact. I remember a silent wait for her body to emerge and then she just appeared, weighing a healthy 7lb (3.2kg). I couldn't believe that both my girls were born with their waters intact. This is seen to be rare but very lucky. I felt so blessed that they were both born safely into the world. We waited for Eryn's cord to stop pulsating and then both girls were returned to me for skin-to-skin. I remember just staring at them, amazed that my birth had gone exactly as I wanted it to. Both girls immediately latched on to feed and I was so proud of them.

After about 45 minutes and having had the injection, I birthed the placenta. I remember being amazed by its size and noticed that both girls' placentas had merged into one giant one. We chose to keep the cords and Tamara had them arranged in a heart shape. Every time I look at them I am reminded of my wonderful twin birth experience. I had no stitches and was told that I could either go home that morning or I could stay on the midwife-led unit for a night. I had a lovely stay with my girls and drove myself home the next morning. Tracey

Unexpected 'free birth'

Choosing the ideal place to give birth is an important decision, but sometimes a baby will arrive in the most unlikely of places. Couples that have done hypnobirthing are often calm and confident about labouring at home. They understand it can take time for a first-time mother's body to find its rhythm and are content at home, only going in to a birthing centre or labour ward when things have progressed rather than early on. This often leads to dads asking in class about what happens if 'baby just shows up!' A birth that isn't attended by medical personnel is known as a 'free birth', and while not encouraging it, Hypnobirthing equips a couple to remain calm and confident wherever their baby decides to join them.

Michelle was planning to be in a birthing centre to welcome her son into the world; he ended up arriving in a far more unusual location!

I was 41+6 days and we had reluctantly agreed to an induction on the Monday (when I'd be 42+2). I had a sweep the night before in a final attempt to get things moving, after trying raspberry leaf tea, acupuncture, curries and the like.

The next day I woke up to a mild period type pain around 6am, but went back to sleep for an hour. Two hours later I started to think something might be happening so ran a bath while listening to the affirmation and rainbow relaxation CD. Richard called the hospital around 9.30am when the surges were 3-4 minutes apart lasting 30-40 seconds and the midwife told us to come in. We had planned to stay at home for as long as possible, but the surges seemed strong with not much recovery time although they were manageable. I felt hazy, internally focussed and relaxed like the women in the hypnobirthing videos I'd seen. The taxi seemed to take forever with our poor cabbie being so considerate about the speed bumps. We got to the assessment ward slowly and gently to be seen by a midwife who examined me at 11am. She told us that I was only 1cm dilated. I was gutted as I felt further along and was only just managing the surges, and now they were sending us home. I wanted to settle and create a safe space. I couldn't face the cab back, only to come back again later. I remembered a story about a doula taking a mum to a hotel to wait through the early stages so we called around to find the nearest hotel, booking into the Radisson Edwardian (the Grafton) on Tottenham Court Road. Checking in, we jokingly promised the nervous receptionist that there was no way we would be giving birth in their hotel.

Once in the room Richard ran a bath and I climbed in, but the surges were so strong I couldn't settle. They were now coming every one to two minutes, but they were only lasting for 30 to 40 seconds. The next position I tried was on the bed, ending up on all fours, and by now I couldn't face light touch massage or any type of physical contact as the gap between the surges was so short. I realised that making noises took the edge off so I was mooing and making the most guttural sounds. I was so worried we'd get complaints from other guests I found myself groaning into the duvet!

At just after 1pm I asked Richard to call the hospital again; by this time I was on all fours in the bathroom wrapped in all the duvets. The midwife heard me in the background and I definitely wasn't calm or serene, but by now we had the CD on loop, which gave me something to focus on. The midwife said it was still too early to come in and suggested I take some paracetamol. I thought I'd got birth all wrong and this was still the early stages of labour. I knew I couldn't go in until I was 4cm dilated and ideally my waters needed to break too. I couldn't comprehend how I could ever do the walk back to the hospital but the CD helped me stay in the moment and I really did feel my primal brain kick in. Richard was amazing; it must have been hard to see me like this but he was calm and supportive. The surges calmed down, which I thought was the paracetamol kicking in – turns out I was in the transition phase. I got calmer and I felt I could go inside myself. I got the urge to push and while I thought it was odd, I went with it as I was keen to get to 4cm so we could get into hospital. A strange thought occurred to me: 'Imagine if I'm having this baby?' It was a concept too good to be true – I still thought I was in the first stages of labour. I was sitting on the loo and I tried to lean forward. I felt the urge to stand and thought I'd put my hand down to check, never thinking it could be my baby, but I could feel the head. 'Rich, I think I'm having this baby', I called. He came in and basically caught the baby.

I looked at him with absolute shock. Did that just happen? I was so relieved, elated and astounded. You hear about these stories but I never thought it would be us. There was our baby, four hours after we'd been turned *away from hospital. Richard called for an ambulance, after making sure I was skin-on-skin with the baby. Six paramedics came to cut the cord and also helped me as I felt quite faint, probably from the shock of it all. I got carried out through reception and into an ambulance back to the hospital to get us both checked out.*

We had a lovely midwife who really took care of us. I delivered the placenta at the hospital but there were concerns that it hadn't all come out. The consultants wanted to put me under general and do an exam but the midwife fought to give it time and for me to have a scan first. We did that and it was all clear so I avoided major intervention after the most natural of births. The hypnobirthing gave me confidence to stand my ground on the care of the baby, specifically around breastfeeding and bonding. I've learnt how to make an informed choice and not get overwhelmed by the professionals and hospital procedure.

I know the story is quite dramatic and I don't want to put anyone off but it was an amazing experience due to the advice and techniques we learnt at hypnobirthing. I am beyond grateful that we signed up, had we not done the course I think our experience would have been traumatic, but instead I feel empowered. I am grateful for the 'mistakes' that were made; had the midwife insisted we come back when we called the second time I would have had to manage the adrenaline of that move. Instead I could stay in my warm dark place with my partner, who was calm and unafraid. I gave birth to a perfect baby boy and feel like a warrior woman. Michelle

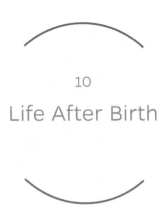

10

Life After Birth

Birth is not only about making babies. Birth is about making mothers – strong, competent, capable mothers who trust themselves and know their inner strength.

Barbara Katz Rothman

Does where, or how we give birth actually matter all that much? The many and frequent debates on this topic often end with the perpetual refrain: 'all that matters is a healthy baby'. Of course a healthy baby and mother are priorities, but it's not *all* that matters. Childbirth affects all involved, emotionally and physically.

Birthrights (a UK organisation committed to improving women's experience of childbirth by promoting respect for human rights) and Mumsnet did a survey in 2013 into women's and midwives' experiences of UK maternity care. They found that the majority of women felt that their experience of childbirth had an impact on their feelings about themselves and their relationships with their babies and partners. A positive impact correlated with spontaneous vaginal births and giving birth in a birth centre. A negative impact correlated strongly with experiencing an instrumental birth. They stated that the impact of childbirth on early motherhood needs to be explored further, with a particular focus on the effects of choice, control and respectful care on women's experiences.

Birth is an emotive subject and hypnobirthing is sometimes accused (by those who don't know much about it) of misleading women, and causing them to feel they've failed if they don't have a natural experience. This sense of succeeding or failing at giving birth is unhelpful and illogical; you cannot be good or bad at giving birth as it is an unconscious act. Because women are terribly self-critical though, if a mother has a bad birth experience at the hands of an overwhelming technocratic system, she often feels in some way responsible and is tormented about whether or not she did the right thing. With thorough antenatal preparation she is able to avoid unnecessary intervention and feel confident and grateful for any help that may be required. Avoiding unnecessary intervention in pregnancy and childbirth has been shown to lead to better outcomes for women; they have a quicker recovery and there is improved satisfaction. Women experiencing a normal birth are more likely to breastfeed, will require less postnatal care and are less likely to visit their doctor with postnatal complications.

After Stella's birth I found I heard a lot more birth stories, and often I was horrified by what I heard. With very few exceptions the majority of people I know who have given birth in hospital have found themselves on a rapidly accelerating medical trajectory, and too many have come away from the experience both physically and emotionally scarred.

Without the inner courage we picked up as a couple from the hypnobirthing I feel sure I would have ended up having an epidural; instead we had a mind-blowing and unique – if physically challenging! – experience in the comfort and security of our own home. I also recovered almost immediately from the birth and I'm sure the positive, can-do attitude was a factor in this too.

Any initial ambivalence about the effectiveness of hypnobirthing on the day has given way entirely to a profound gratitude that Oliver and I went into the birth excited, relaxed and confident that we were together equipped to make the right decisions for me and Stella. Hypnobirthing helped me to silence the anxious, whispering voices and take control of my beautiful baby's birthing. Mary

There is emerging scientific evidence linking our current birthing practices to the increased risk of our children developing non-communicable diseases such as heart disease, some cancers, asthma and diabetes. Scientists are only just beginning to understand the microbiome – the unique colony of microbial organisms that populates every human – and they're looking into the role it plays, not just in birth, but in every aspect of our mental and physical health. The studies are indicating that if we encourage natural physiological birth where possible, with full support for immediate skin-to-skin contact and breastfeeding, then that baby has the best possible chance of a healthy immune system.

Why is this? Well when the baby emerges, it is entering a world of bacteria, some of which are bad but some of which are good. In the weeks and days leading up to birth, specific species of good bacteria are migrating to key locations in the mother's body and are transferred to the baby during and immediately after birth via the birth path, immediate skin-to-skin contact and breastfeeding. The role of these good bacteria is to train the baby's human cells to distinguish between what is 'friend' and what is 'foe', so that its immune system can fight off attack from pathogens. This process kickstarts the baby's immune system and helps to protect the infant from disease for its entire lifetime.

So babies born vaginally are colonised with friendly microbes, good familiar microbes. This is how it's been for generations; you could say our human system has been educated this way. However, with interventions like the use of synthetic oxytocin, antibiotics, c-section and formula feeding, this microbial transfer from the mother to baby is interfered with or bypassed completely. Studies comparing the microbiomes of vaginally born babies with those born via caesarean have shown differences in their gut bacteria as much as seven years after birth. There is much we don't yet understand about why or how much these differences may matter, but pregnancy, birth and breastfeeding 'seed' our microbiome and therefore have a long-term effect on health.

On an even wider scale, could it be that our birth choices are making fundamental differences to our babies, and therefore matter to the whole human race, in deeply important ways? Could the way we are giving birth even be altering our entire direction, as a species? There are many experts who believe so.

Until recently an intense activation of the oxytocin system was needed to bring the baby, but the number of women now giving birth to their baby and placenta with this cocktail of love hormones is diminishing. The increase in induced labours and caesarean section birth means that women don't need or use their own natural hormones. We still don't know what the long-term effects of this will be. Is there not a risk, though, that the human oxytocin system will become weaker and weaker? Let's not forget the role that natural oxytocin plays in our lives, in childbirth, in breastfeeding, in sex, in all aspects of love and empathy for our fellow human beings. We could be altering future generations without knowing it. Michel Odent, in his book *Childbirth and the Evolution of Homo Sapiens* argues that 'One cannot go on creating massive disturbances in childbirth and breastfeeding without altering the sexual life and the capacity to love of society as a whole.'

When we're talking about this kind of epidemiological research (epidemiology meaning the study of disease and health in *populations*), please remember we are not talking about any single individual. This is not about just you or the people you know, this is about our global human family, and our shared future as a species. Our increased understanding of the importance of the environment around and within a birthing mother, rather than creating feelings of anxiety about 'getting it right', will hopefully act as a catalyst for both expectant parents and health care providers to provide it. The potential benefits to us all cannot be underestimated. As Katharine Graves of KG Hypnobirthing says:

> *Women come to hypnobirthing for the best birth for them, and it certainly delivers. But if birth is calm, more comfortable, and drug free for you, it is also calm, more comfortable and drug free for your baby. When a baby who enters the world this way, to be greeted by a mother who is ready to receive it in an alert and gentle state, this is how it forms its first relationship in this world. This is the blueprint for every relationship it forms throughout its life, so it will affect it throughout its life, and will even affect all the people it meets. Our world needs more people like this, and the importance of this cannot be over-estimated.*

Hypnobirthing after birth

There is a lot of energy and excitement after a baby is born and in this day of Facebook and Twitter, instant messaging and emails, there's a temptation to shout the news from the rooftops and want to share your excitement with everyone. Those first few days and weeks with your newborn are sacred, however, and will lay the foundations for this next chapter in your life.

Becoming a mother is probably the most life-changing experience any woman goes through. Conceiving, growing and birthing a baby is really a year-long physical process (longer for those who have been trying to conceive for some time) and it takes time for a woman's body to recover, heal and settle after giving birth. The concept of a 'babymoon', a planned period of calm spent together by a just-born baby and its parents, is well known and many cultures recognise this with a period of 'lying-in' where the tradition is to care for a mother and her baby for the first forty days or so after birth, so she need not cook, clean, or otherwise leave her baby's side. These cultures understand the importance of healing and bonding after the birth, but in the West we have lost this, pressurising women to get 'back to normal' as soon as possible after birth. In minimising the time they need to recover from the birth and get to know their babies, we trivialise the event. Not surprising then that 10 per cent of women in the UK have severe postnatal depression and many more feel they 'can't cope'. We need to rediscover the art of mothering the new mother.

Newborns cannot fend for themselves and still have much developing to do – they completely rely on you for every single need. A gentle adjustment into their new world in this time of a 'babymoon' or 'fourth trimester', as it's increasingly becoming known, can make a huge difference to how baby feels and how mum and dad cope with parenthood. Studies have shown that babies who receive plenty of skin-to-skin contact are more likely to latch on to the breast well, breastfeed exclusively and for a longer period of time, have a stable temperature and a normal heart rate and blood pressure, have higher blood sugar, are less likely to cry, and will self-wake when they are hungry.

So whether you have a home or hospital birth, the first few days and weeks at home are a chance for you to take full advantage of your newborn's sleepy state and rest in bed with them, letting your body heal while you hold and pamper your baby with love. These days returning to modern life means obeying other rhythms than those of your baby and delaying that return will yield great benefits for both you and your baby.

A week after I gave birth, I noticed my left-brain activity returning. I felt a sort of mourning for that pregnancy state of consciousness because I noticed that left-brain processes were accompanied by a background anxiety created by thinking once again about the past and the future. This is when I fully realised the beauty and wonder of that special opportunity of pregnancy consciousness. To access that state again, I knew I would have to practise meditation or live in the present moment with my baby as a kind of living meditation. This requires more intention or effort than being gifted inner birthing wisdom in pregnancy by Mother Nature.
Amali Lokugamage *The Heart In The Womb*

Dr Lokugamage describes how pregnancy can naturally bring a woman into that state of 'no brain': the cynical among us deride 'pregnancy brain' as a bad thing, whereas it's actually your clever instinct encouraging you away from your neo-cortex in preparation for birth! Continuing the practice of stepping away from your 'thinking brain' after giving birth requires effort, but the health benefits are enormous. Hypnosis has been shown to rejuvenate, replenish and heal the body and mind. It can boost the immune system, reduce stress and anxiety and improve sleep. The deep rest brought about through hypnosis allows you to tap into your infinite energy reserves, which is so helpful when your sleep patterns are disturbed by a newborn wanting to be fed in the middle of the night.

As a new parent your sympathetic nervous system will go into overdrive as the protective instinct kicks in for your newborn; suddenly leaving the house and crossing the road seems fraught with danger. With hypnobirthing preparation, however, you're already well-versed in recognising symptoms of the stress response and have the tools to quickly return to a state of balance.

Just as there is no one right way to birth, there is no right way to parent. Hypnobirthing teaches a couple to tune into and to trust their instincts, which is crucial as you learn who your child is and what kind of parent you want to be. The hypnobirthing approach you adopt through pregnancy serves you well in this new chapter in your life, and it can affect the way you parent and the adults your children grow into.

If you want to optimise your health, extend your life expectancy, and feel as vital as possible, you need to help your nervous system live in a state of peace. Hypnobirthing teaches you exactly this approach. Ideally we can learn to live, for the most part, in a baseline state of calm peacefulness with mild stress responses for enthusiasm, vitality, wholesome passions, and occasional spikes to deal with demanding situations. This could well be your best-odds prescription for a long, productive, happy life!

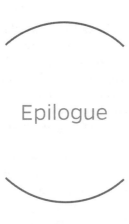

Epilogue

While we can prove the benefits of leaving birth alone, there is still something of a cultural blindness to the ramifications of current birth practice. The conditions conducive to normal birth are well known and yet often not provided. Society, including the medical world, remains blind to the science so we must rely on counter-cultural ways of thinking to herald a new era of bringing babies calmly into the world.

In a backlash against the medicalisation of birth women are beginning to reclaim their experience of pregnancy and birth and a counter-culture has emerged. Film, images and stories of empowered birthing mothers circulate through the internet – women birthing in beautiful environments looking powerful, in control, focused and calm. Women are able to see how birth can be, and many are inspired and driven to create a birth experience like those they watch.

Women are the experts in their own bodies and babies and, given full information, they will make the choices that are right for them and their babies, whether that's in line with what their friends, family and current medical practice is saying or not. When an idea reaches critical mass, what was the idea of a few people suddenly becomes everybody's idea. One woman tells another, and soon a hundred people have heard about hypnobirthing. Each birth creates a ripple effect in the community – it's amazing the effect that a normal birth has on people.

If you're an expectant parent reading this, I hope I've encouraged you to consider hypnobirthing as a way of preparing for this new chapter in your life. It's the little decisions that make a big impact down the line. Picking up a book about hypnobirthing now may seem like a little decision, but it can certainly have a big impact down the line when you meet your baby...

To all the birthing partners, midwives, doulas and birth workers, I salute you and thank you for your support, wisdom and enthusiasm. When we're all working together to create a safe, supportive space for the birthing mother anything is possible. To all the mothers, you are more powerful than you know and I wish you and your babies a calm, confident and joyous birth.

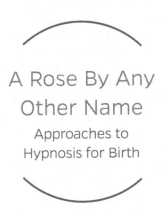

A Rose By Any Other Name

Approaches to
Hypnosis for Birth

KG Hypnobirthing
created by Katharine Graves

Is KG Hypnobirthing possible with self-study? Would you advise parents-to-be to attend classes?

Many people ask me if the book and CDs are sufficient to do KG Hypnobirthing, and the honest answer is, 'I don't know!' For some it will be sufficient, and others need to come to a class, and there is no way of telling which category a woman comes into until she has had her baby.

How long is a KG Hypnobirthing course for expectant couples?

Hypnobirthing is a full 12-hour training. Some people offer short courses and, indeed, you can teach the techniques in a shorter time, but this is to miss the point. Hypnobirthing is far more than a few techniques to apply in labour. You need an understanding of how and why hypnobirthing works so well in order for it to be most effective. You also need an understanding of how it fits into 'the system' and how best to get the best out of 'the system'. People have come to my classes having done a shorter course and feeling they hadn't really 'got it', and then realised that they needed the full course.

There is no research or evidence that one format for a class is better than another, though some people hold strong views on this. I have taught in all formats, five short sessions, four short sessions, two full days in separate weekends, and two full days in the same weekend. Each format has its benefits. The argument for four or five evenings is that there is plenty of time to practise in between. The disadvantages are that pregnant women are almost falling off their chairs with tiredness when they have already done a day's work. The argument for full days is that you build up a wonderful group rapport, you are fresh, and it's easier to fit in to a busy life. To do it in two weekends gives you time to absorb the information in between. To do it in one weekend builds up a fantastic group rapport. I have taught it in all formats and my observation is that it works perfectly well in any format, so it is best to do the one that fits in with your lifestyle.

What training do qualified teachers of KG Hypnobirthing receive?
The KG Hypnobirthing Teacher Training course consists of three modules, each of two days:

- Hypnotherapy for Hypnobirthing (exemption if you are already trained in hypnotherapy, NLP, etc.),
- Hypnobirthing Teacher Training
- Birthing Foundation (exemption if you are a midwife, doula, NCT teacher, etc.)

This equips a Hypnobirthing Teacher to fully understand all aspects of how and what they are teaching, rather than teaching by rote. All the trainers are qualified hypnobirthing teachers with particular qualifications in their area of expertise. For example, the hypnotherapy module is always taught by a qualified hypnotherapist, and the Birthing Foundation module is taught by a qualified midwife. The Hypnobirthing Teacher Training module is taught by a very experienced hypnobirthing teacher, often Katharine Graves herself, and if not Katharine, by someone she has personally trained. Someone training in hypnobirthing wants to be sure they are being taught by an expert in what the student has come to learn. If you are already a hypnotherapist you want to learn from someone with a different area of expertise as you have the hypnotherapy knowledge already. If you are a midwife you also want to be taught by someone with a different area of expertise as you have the midwifery knowledge already.

Is the training recognised by any professional bodies?
The KG Hypnobirthing Teacher Training course is accredited by the Royal College of Midwives (RCM), the highest accolade a course can receive. KG Hypnobirthing is also a member of FEDANT.

Would you say there is a particular emphasis with KG Hypnobirthing that other hypnosis for birth courses perhaps don't have?
The principles on which all hypnobirthing courses are based are the same. A principle has universal application and is immutable. KG Hypnobirthing not only empowers you to achieve a calm and comfortable birth, but it also gives you uniquely the tools to get the best out of the system in which you find yourself. The medical world often presents routine procedures as the only way, or the only safe way, of giving birth. KG Hypnobirthing helps you to understand what your options are, what the repercussions of any proposed procedures are likely to be, and how to work with your

medical advisers to achieve the best birth for you. When you understand the logic of how hypnobirthing works – why it works so well – then you can apply what you are taught with maximum effect to achieve a calm and more comfortable birth for you – and for your baby.

Mindful Mamma
created by Sophie Fletcher

Is Mindful Mamma possible with self-study? Would you advise parents-to-be to attend classes?
I think you can do a certain amount of self-study. However, hypnotherapy is principally about processing unconscious anxieties and fears, and this can only really be done in a practitioner-led, structured way. The support of a practitioner in reflection and learning techniques can also increase confidence in using them. When my second child was born, and before I trained, my experience was of listening to MP3s without a class or book. It did a great job but only took me so far. I often think that had I had a course or practitioner to learn from I would have made different choices, and perhaps been more assertive.

How long is a Mindful Mamma course for expectant couples?
I've thought long and hard about this. I've taught classes in twelve hours, six hours and two hours. I found that there was little difference in outcomes between twelve hours and six hours, but massive differences between two and six. I find six hours works really well. With Mindful Mamma we teach just hypnosis and mindfulness, we don't cover much physiology. This is all covered in the book, *Mindful Hypnobirthing*, which means we are able to teach the essentials you would need in addition to a book – so our focus is on practical techniques

and interactive learning. This is great for busy parents who want to just do a class and get on with the practice. At the end of the day it's all about changing beliefs, letting go of fear and conditioning responses. You don't need hours and hours of tuition to do this. All you need to do is learn the principles, commit yourself to practise every day and your body will respond really well. As a hypnotherapist I see people change beliefs, learn self-hypnosis or shift phobias and anxieties in as little as an hour, and while I'm not saying you can do a hypnobirthing course in an hour, it does demonstrate how fast it works as an intervention.

What training do qualified teachers of Mindful Mamma receive?
We are slightly different to others in this and it's why we are also a lot smaller. We only train people who are midwives, or talking therapists – everyone who trains already has extensive experience of working with women psychologically. This means I am absolutely confident in the quality of classes being delivered and I know it sounds boring, but I think an inherent understanding of ethical boundaries is vital to keep women safe. I know that each one of my practitioners has solid training and understanding of this because of their background. This means our training is shorter, it's more like Continuing Professional Development (CPD). All practitioners learn the course and have an additional six hours in delivering hypnosis maternity training, as well as a marketing module. If they are a hypnotherapist they will get a basic natal physiology course of six hours.

Is the training recognised by any professional bodies?
We haven't applied for any recognition for the course itself. We regard it more an extension of our practitioners' existing professional practice. As a result each of our practitioners is registered with a Department of Health recognised body in their

own right and, as they are able to tailor courses based on their own professional background, it keeps safe and well-supervised structures in place for their work with women and their partners.

Would you say there is a particular emphasis with Mindful Mammas that other hypnosis for birth courses perhaps don't have? I view our course philosophy as slightly different to others. Our focus isn't just hypnosis, we also look at current evidence-based work around the psychology of birth, why expectations and belief affect experience of sensations or pain, and unconscious emotional and physical responses to our environment that make birth harder. We also explore the interaction of hypnosis and mindfulness as interventions during birth. The philosophy is about creating the perfect environment internally and externally for birth to flourish. When this happens women's bodies can do it. Of course we teach hypnosis techniques to be used at different stages in labour, but the message is that when you go into labour 100 per cent trusting in the process and your body you don't need hypnosis, you don't need anything apart from good support and to be present in each moment – that's the mindfulness element. We teach very specific mindfulness techniques. More unusually we teach the partners about mindfulness and the importance of setting their own judgements aside during the birth.

We wanted to create a class that was adaptable, evidence-based and practical. We don't teach what you can read in a book; our class is based on interactive learning. One quote from a dad that sums it up is, 'it tells you what's happening, why it happens and what (or not) to do about it'.

HypnoBirthing – The Mongan Method
created by Marie Mongan

Sonia Richards and Steve Griffiths are the longest serving practitioners of The Mongan Method in the UK, are members of the HypnoBirthing Advisory Board for the UK & Ireland and are responding here as representatives of the HypnoBirthing Institute.

Is HypnoBirthing – The Mongan Method possible with self-study? Would you advise parents-to-be to attend classes?
The short answer is that self-study will only work for a few highly motivated people. I have known people who have bought the book and a CD who have attempted self-study with mixed results. Those who already possess strong positive beliefs in themselves and nature's way of birthing are more likely to achieve this. I'm sure that you can guess that the numbers of women birthing in our current fear-filled, medicalised climate with those firm beliefs in place are extremely small. For the majority of women self-study is not going to be enough to dispel fears and concerns. A book or CD cannot build as much confidence, answer questions, demonstrate techniques first-hand and be there to observe when women and their birthing companions are practising those techniques.

HypnoBirthing classes are incredibly good value for money. We cover all aspects of antenatal education including physiological functions in pregnancy and birth, nutrition, positions for labour and birth, special circumstances when nature may need assistance, practicalities of birthing at home, birthing centre or hospital, water birth, information on Vitamin K, birth plans, perineal massage, exercise, what interventions are and how to avoid them, safe natural ways to encourage the body towards labour, support requirements during labour, what to expect immediately after birthing, birthing the placenta, bonding both pre- and postnatal, information on breastfeeding and the role of companions or assistants such as doulas.

Equally as important, clients get the support of a Professional HypnoBirthing Childbirth Educator who in many cases is also a Clinical Hypnotherapist and Complementary Therapist who may also have a medical background and perhaps be a midwife or doula. This on-going support is key to women maintaining the positive mindset created in the classes throughout their own daily practice.

How long is a Mongan Method HypnoBirthing course for expectant couples?
The minimum requirement in order to fully cover the syllabus and allow for practice of techniques within the class is twelve and a half hours. Ideally five sessions is the minimum; this can vary if the woman comes to classes later than 35 weeks into her pregnancy or lives a long distance from her nearest practitioner.

We are effectively creating a new positive habit to default the mind to birth being a normal, natural physiological event in normal, healthy women carrying normal, healthy babies. Little and often, and repetition is the key to reprogramming and getting rid of old faulty or negative beliefs. Trying to cram at least twelve and a half hours of information, education and techniques into a few days can be a lot to ask anyone to assimilate, let alone a pregnant woman whose metabolism and brain function has changed quite significantly. A fair amount of the teaching will be missed because the mind distorts, deletes and generalises information and sensory input all of the time. Also seeing a couple over several weeks helps build rapport and a relationship of trust, as well as constant, positive reaffirmation of normality and that birth can indeed be a comfortable and joyous event.

What training do qualified teachers of HypnoBirthing – The Mongan Method receive?

Training has changed from the original criteria when only hypnotherapists were allowed to train. We now include midwives, other talking therapy modalities, complementary therapies, medical professionals, doulas and even HypnoBirthing mothers who have had a wonderful HypnoBirthing experience.

Depending on the level of experience there are different training routes available. Those with no hypnosis experience who are not working within the birthing profession must complete the Hypnosis module as well as the Birth Basics module and HypnoBirthing Programme training. Those with both (i.e. a midwife who is also a hypnotherapist) can train purely in delivering the programme, although many still choose to do the home study Birth Basics module as a form of Continual Professional Development (CPD). Hypnotherapists with no birthing background must complete the Birth Basics module as taught by a HypnoBirthing midwife prior to the HypnoBirthing Programme training.

On completion of the training, case studies are performed in which clients are not charged to attend classes; a written exam review must be completed and if this is not successfully answered further training may be required.

The HypnoBirthing Institute requires all Practitioners to perform CPD in order to recertify every year. This can include giving talks or university lectures, writing articles, reading books or further training in the field of birthing and hypnosis and other therapeutic modalities. The Institute has a wide-ranging programme of further training such as HypnoBirthing Doula Certification, HypnoMothering, HypnoBirthing Fertility Therapist, HypnoBirthing Baby Massage Therapist, HypnoParenting, and HypnoBirthing Support Techniques for

Birth Workers. Hence it is ever-evolving and improving the services offered to parents and professionals.

Is it recognised by any professional bodies?
It is recognised by all of the major hypnotherapy professional bodies in most of the countries where it operates. e.g. National Guild of Hypnotists in the USA, General Hypnotherapy Register in the UK. It is also recognised by FEDANT.

Would you say there is a particular emphasis with HypnoBirthing – The Mongan Method that other hypnosis for birth courses perhaps don't have?
I would say one main emphasis is the belief that starting as early into the pregnancy as possible has a really positive effect on the emotional and physical wellbeing of mother and baby. More classes also help to build relationships between the practitioner and clients and increase the support both before and after birth.

We also have the advantage of 25 years of evidence to back up our results, after the personal experience of the founder Marie Mongan, who used similar techniques for her own birthings, then created this programme for her daughter and grandson Kyle, the first official HypnoBirthing baby born in the world!

Natal Hypnotherapy
created by Maggie Howell

Is Natal Hypnotherapy possible with self-study?
Yes, it was all I used for the birth of my first son in 2000 and it worked so incredibly well that I went on to create Natal Hypnotherapy as a self-hypnosis, home-use programme to help reduce any fear around childbirth, to learn to fully relax and to build confidence. As I started to see more women in my private hypnotherapy practice, I realised that my CD for home birth

was not applicable to women choosing a hospital birth and so I created more for births in hospital and birth centres, VBACs, caesarean and twin births and for pre- and post-birth.

I recommend women start listening to the CDs as early as possible in their pregnancy to get maximum benefit. It teaches fundamental relaxation and breathing techniques with visualisations and suggestions which are applicable to pregnancy; they can then move onto the Birth Preparation CDs from around 32 weeks.

In 2009 I brought out my *Effective Birth Preparation* book as an accompaniment to the CDs. The book was the accumulation of all I had learnt and developed working with women individually as well as during our classes. The CDs and book are accessible and affordable so we are able to reach a higher number of women than those choosing to attend a class. Approximately 70 per cent of all women who have used Natal Hypnotherapy have just used the CDs and book.

Would you advise parents-to-be to attend classes?
Ideally all parents would have access to this kind of birth preparation. However, currently it is more for those couples that can afford it, or for those who view birth preparation as a priority over other expenses. Although the CDs are the foundation to the Natal Hypnotherapy approach, the classes teach couples, especially the birth partner, so much more. There are two one-day classes available – one on 'Natural Pain Relief' and the other on 'Practical Birth Preparation'.

The classes teach more in-depth birth preparation skills with a wide range of practical, informative tools and techniques to help the mother and her birth partner feel more confident and prepared for birth. These include an easy to understand guide to what will happen in labour, managing the emotional states in labour, pain management techniques, rapid triggers to enter hypnosis, massage, visualisation, using your breath effectively, working with the medical team, personalising your birth suggestions, and tools for the birth partner to help keep the mother calm and relaxed. They are no longer frightened about the experience and so find that they enjoy practising the techniques, take time out to relax, and let go of all the old fears and concerns. At the end of each workshop, couples leave feeling confident, excited and truly prepared.

How long is a Natal Hypnotherapy course for expectant couples?
The majority of Natal Hypnotherapy classes are run over two full days totalling fourteen hours. Some practitioners run them over four evening classes or half-day sessions, but the content and hours are the same.

What training do qualified teachers of Natal Hypnotherapy receive?
All potential trainees go through an application and interview process prior to being accepted on the training course with limited places available. This is to ensure that the quality of our practitioners remains consistently high and that they each share the same passion, beliefs and ethos of Natal Hypnotherapy.

Practitioners are taught life skills, coaching and facilitation skills and many find the rigorous and intense training a life-changing experience. In addition to the five-day training, they attend a two-day assessment, which gives them the opportunity to run through the whole weekend with 'real couples' in a safe and nurtured setting with the mentorship of either myself or one of my senior assessors. This also ensures that all practitioners are teaching the Natal Hypnotherapy course to the same consistently high standard. Once trained there is an ongoing mentorship support programme to ensure that new practitioners have the confidence, knowledge and support to run successful classes.

Is it recognised by any professional bodies?
Yes, it was accredited by the Royal College of Midwives in 2013.

Would you say there is a particular emphasis with Natal Hypnotherapy that other hypnosis for birth courses perhaps don't have?
All the different approaches are using the same principles and have the same goal in mind – to empower women to have better births – but I feel that Natal Hypnotherapy is different on a few levels.

The CDs and book are the fundamental part of the approach, rather than the courses. I have had thousands of birth stories from women having amazing, empowering births from just listening to the CDs. The Natal Hypnotherapy approach is truly based on giving birth in the UK maternity system. The classes have continued to evolve and change according to the latest guidelines and the content in the classes reflects the environment that women will be giving birth in. Thirdly, the classes are tailored to each individual. Each couple is given personalised suggestions, affirmations and triggers. During hypnosis sessions, each person is given very specific suggestions to help them with their own personal issues.

Women are not led to believe that birth, if done correctly, will be pain free, or that there is a right or wrong way of breathing etc. Women are encouraged to accept all sensations and to work with them. Also we do not encourage women to change common words such as contraction to 'surge' or to not use words such as 'pain'. Instead we focus on helping the mother to have confidence and trust in her own ability no matter what is going on around her.

The Wise Hippo Birthing Programme
created by Dany Griffiths

Is The Wise Hippo Birthing Programme possible with self-study? Would you advise parents-to-be to attend classes?
No. We believe that it is possible to learn hypnobirthing successfully without attending classes, but there is so much more to be gained by doing so, including motivation and inspiration from instructors, along with the confidence gained from knowing that they are understanding correctly through being able to question and clarify.

We find that although some couples initially think that it will be hard to find time to attend a course, they are sad when it comes to an end. They have enjoyed dedicating the time to preparing well for their baby's birth, as well as the bonding time together and with their baby. For many finding time for this is often the hardest thing to achieve in their modern-day busy lives. Many couples also enjoy meeting others socially and establishing friendships along the way.

How long is a Wise Hippo course for expectant couples?
The course totals ten hours and is ideally run as four 2.5-hour sessions, although we leave it to the instructor and client to decide what is best for them, based on time and location. Some instructors do the course as two 5-hour sessions, although unless time and location make it very difficult we recommend that this is not done over a weekend. We like to see how the couple are progressing and this is obviously more achievable when the course sessions are spread out.

Instructors also provide continuous support via phone and email and The Wise Hippo has an online chat group which also helps our clients meet other like-minded couples. They can also ask questions of any of our instructor community who have a vast range of additional skills and knowledge. We can of course also all celebrate with them when their babies are born.

What training do qualified teachers of Wise Hippo receive?
We have a foundation level for Birth and Hypnosis. Trainees will complete the ones relevant to them based on their current experience/qualifications. The main instructor training covers three key areas:

- How to teach The Wise Hippo Birthing Programme.
- Teaching skills.
- How to get started with their businesses, marketing and how to prepare for their case study. We make sure that they are ready to 'hit the ground running'.

The final assessment is a case study. The trainee will self-evaluate on a number of key criteria, eg how they prepared, how they felt prior, during and post training, their timing, what they did well, what they could do better, their 'client's' reactions and questions, etc. The 'client' will also evaluate their performance.

There are no previous qualifications required to become a Wise Hippo instructor but we do highly recommend that individuals have a passion for wanting to help pregnant couples.

We also provide continuous support via phone and our online chat group, which is a great resource for instructors to have any questions answered quickly.

Is it recognised by any professional bodies?
It was granted accreditation by the RCM in 2014 and is recognised by FEDANT.

Would you say there is a particular emphasis with The Wise Hippo that other hypnosis for birth courses perhaps don't have?
We believe a 'positive birth' experience is a state of mind; it's not defined by what happens during labour and birth, but by how a woman feels about her baby's birth. Because of this belief we are able to teach skills and knowledge that empower women to trust their instincts and ensure that their baby has the right birth on the day.

We respect that every woman has the right to choose the birth that she wants for her child (whatever that may be) and we trust that our clients know what is right for them. We therefore don't tell our clients what they 'should' do, we don't offer advice and we don't give them our personal opinion.

There is no one right way to give birth with The Wise Hippo, only the right way for each individual mum and her baby. The Wise Hippo is non-partisan and suitable for all, including mothers without partners and same-sex couples.

What we do is provide our clients with a fun programme full of factual information about labour and birth, along with simple to follow tools and techniques, so that they are able to alleviate any fears, build their confidence. become experts in relaxation and ensure that they are always the ones in control of their baby's birth (whatever turn their birthing takes).

Our clients leave our courses feeling excited, empowered and confident that they have the skills to remain calm, relaxed and in control throughout their labour and birth no matter what path it takes.

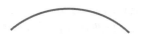

Further Reading and Resources

KG Hypnobirthing *The Hypnobirthing Book* by Katharine Graves kghypnobirthing.com

Mindful Mamma *Mindful HypnoBirthing* by Sophie Fletcher mindfulmamma.co.uk

The Mongan Method *HypnoBirthing* by Marie Mongan hypnobirthing.co.uk

Natal Hypnotherapy *Effective Birth Preparation* by Maggie Howell natalhypnotherapy.co.uk

The Wise Hippo thewisehippo.com

Books about birth

Gentle Birth, Gentle Mothering by Sarah Buckley (Celestial Arts, 2009) Evidence-based work that can support your birth preferences, or encourage you to think about alternatives.

Childbirth Without Fear by Grantly Dick-Read (Pinter & Martin, 2013) The book that arguably started it all.

Bump: How to Make, Grow and Birth a Baby by Kate Evans

(Myriad Editions, 2014). Straightforward, funny and accessible, with detailed laugh-out-loud cartoons that demystify the complexities of pregnancy and birth.

Ina May's Guide to Childbirth by Ina May Gaskin (Vermilion, 2008) The book that most mums say changed their view of birth.

Spiritual Midwifery by Ina May Gaskin (4th Ed, Book Publishing Company, 2002) Especially for the midwives and birth workers among you.

The Heart In The Womb by Amali Lokugamage (Docamali, 2011) Written by a consultant obstetrician at a London hospital, this explores what risk and decision-making really mean.

Primal Health by Michel Odent (Clairview Books, 2007) Explores how the period between conception and a child's first birthday is critical to life-long health.

Childbirth and the Evolution of Homo Sapiens by Michel Odent (Pinter & Martin, 2014) Asks questions about the impact of intervention in birth for the future of our species.

Birth & Sex by Sheila Kitzinger (Pinter & Martin, 2012) Explores the complexity and depth of female sexuality during pregnancy, birth, and after the baby comes.

Books for dads recommended by dads

Commando Dad: Raw Recruits: from pregnancy to birth by Neil Sinclair (Yellow Kite, 2014) Loosely based on the British Army's Basic Battle Skills, this a fun but ultimately useful book for every man about to embark on his greatest ever mission: fatherhood.

Pregnancy for men – the whole nine months by Mark Woods (White Ladder Press, 2010) From how your baby grows month-by-month, to how to support your partner.

Men, Love & Birth: the book about being present at birth that your pregnant lover wants you to read by Mark Harris (Pinter & Martin, 2015).

Support for expectant parents and birth workers during pregnancy and birth

AIMS – The Association for Improvement in Maternity Services aims.org.uk – A UK charity with a wide range of publications about pregnancy and birth – all are highly recommended. They are available in paperback and e-book from the AIMS website.

Birthrights – birthrights.org.uk – A UK organisation founded by a group of lawyers committed to improving women's experience of childbirth by promoting respect for human rights. They have insightful fact sheets on their website and support mothers and midwives.

IMUK - Independent Midwives UK – imuk.org.uk – IMUK is the membership organisation for independent midwives in the UK offering support for women with the very best evidence-based care and helping to safeguard authentic midwifery both in and out of the NHS.

Other useful websites and blogs

sarahbuckley.com – Sarah Buckley is a doctor and author who writes wonderfully on all aspects of pregnancy and birth.

sarawickham.com – A midwife, researcher and author whose site contains hundreds of free articles and blog posts for anyone seeking information about birth and midwifery.

midwifethinking.com – Midwife Rachel Reed writes eloquently and with evidence-based care about all things pregnancy and birth.

tellmeagoodbirthstory.com – Lots of amazing birth stories, inspirational and informational.

positivebirthmovement.org – Local groups helping support women to have positive births all over the world.

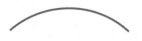

Acknowledgements

I'm so grateful to Susan Last and Martin Wagner at Pinter & Martin for the opportunity to share my passion and hopefully help a wider audience understand just how powerful hypnosis is for everyone welcoming babies into the world.

Many thanks to all the hypnobirthing teachers and course creators who contributed their time: Katharine Graves at KG Hypnobirthing, Marie Mongan, Sonia Richards and Steve Griffiths at the HypnoBirthing Institute, Sophie Fletcher at Mindful Mamma, Maggie Howell at Natal Hypnotherapy and Dany Griffiths and Tamara Ciamfini at The Wise Hippo.

Also to fellow hypnobirthing teachers who shared stories: Jacqueline A. Grimsley, Ruth Sabrosa, Lucy Atkinson and Chris Ojari.

I'm so grateful to those who not only inspire me but also generously contributed and brainstormed with me and also checked what I was writing made sense: Milli Hill at the Positive Birth Movement, Jacqui, Elke, Mal and Anna from the London Birth Practice, Vanessa Hodge, Dr Amali Lokugamage, Mark Harris, Elizabeth Prochaska at Birthrights and Beverly Harper at Calming Mind. I am indebted to the talented 'womb artist' Clare Wilson who was able, at the very last minute, to convey exactly what was in my head on the page.

I know how powerful it is to hear of others' experiences, so much gratitude to all the wonderful 'hypnobirthers' who generously shared their experiences with me: Corinne de Alwis, Michelle Booth, Kat Butterfield, Maya Carni, Richard Delaney, Claudia Draper, Manuela Ferrigni, Amy Fleming, Tracey Harper, Sophie Hilton, Kathryn Kramer, Isobel Martin, Anna Phoebe, Anna Sudbury, Rick Sellers, Mary Stevens, Ellie Taylor and Carly Walker Smith.

A very special thank you to those close to me who have always encouraged and supported me, believing in me when I doubted myself. Love you MORE especially to Momma Bear, to my sister Jo who selflessly sat by a pool reading chapters and to my comrade Claire, who could have had no idea that by inviting me to her beautiful boys' births she would contribute so hugely to changing my life; Billy and Sam you give the best hugs!

Finally to all those I've shared hypnobirthing with over the years and to those I'll meet in the future; it's truly a privilege to share this exciting time with you and to learn and understand more with each of you. Every baby is unique and so is their birth. The miraculous force of nature and the grace and power of a birthing woman never ceases to amaze me and I wish for you all a joyous, peaceful pregnancy and a calm and confident birth.

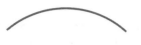

Index